9
10.7.08

The New Reflexology

The New Reflexology

A Unique Blend of Traditional Chinese Medicine
and Western Reflexology Practice for Better
Health and Healing

Inge Dougans

Marlowe & Company • New York

THE NEW REFLEXOLOGY:
A Unique Blend of Traditional Chinese Medicine and
Western Reflexology Practice for Better Health and Healing

Copyright © 2006 by Inge Dougans

Published by
Marlowe & Company
An Imprint of Avalon Publishing Group, Incorporated
245 West 17th Street • 11th floor
New York, NY 10011

AVALON
publishing group incorporated

This edition was published in somewhat different form in 2005 in Great Britain under the title *Reflexology* by Thorsons, an imprint of HarperCollins Publishers.
This edition is published by arrangement with Thorsons.

Library of Congress Cataloging-in-Publication Data is available.

ISBN: 1-56924-289-5
ISBN-13: 978-1-56924-289-6

9 8 7 6 5 4 3 2 1

Printed in the United States of America

contents

introduction

Over the last two decades, reflexology has become an established form of natural healing that is now gaining wide acceptance in the Western world. Yet reflexology has grown out of a much older system: traditional Chinese Medicine (TCM).

The practice of TCM, including acupuncture, goes back several thousand years. Since that time it has been well preserved and continuously developed. TCM is characterized by its specific diagnostic techniques and therapeutic principles based on a practitioner's interpretation of the physiological functions and pathological changes in the human body.

Reflexology also works on pressure points to stimulate the body's own healing potential, but mainly in the feet and with specific massage techniques. Even though reflexology has its roots in ancient Eastern forms of healing, the development of modern reflexology has happened primarily in the West. When reflexology first emerged in the West, the traditional Chinese energy pathways, or meridians, and the associated pressure points in the body were not common knowledge. As a result, reflexologists independently developed their interpretations of energy zones in the body and corresponding pressure points.

The ten reflexology zones are helpful, but we can gain a greater understanding of the energy pathways in the body if we look to TCM.

I have been practising and teaching reflexology for over 25 years. These years of experience have made it clear to me that elements of traditional Chinese Medicine can – and indeed should – play a vital role in the effective practice of reflexology. For example, when you work with a patient to assess the root cause of an ailment or condition, the Chinese meridian system is more accurate than the ten reflexology zones. It is time for reflexology to revisit its Eastern roots and draw vital lessons from its ancient heritage to enhance its practice.

There is another essential part of reflexology training I advocate that is not a part of traditional reflexology training: diet. Reflexology, like many of the natural healing therapies available today, cannot be successfully applied without also considering how the body is nourished. What we eat has a profound impact on the general environment of the body and also affects how well it can respond to healing treatments. If a person has poor eating habits it will make congestions and diseases denser and more difficult for the body to eliminate. This is why you must also look at a person's diet as part of their overall treatment, in particular their blood sugar and acid–alkaline balance, since a body that is too acid is more vulnerable to disease and injury. If you take steps to establish a healthy environment in the body it is much easier to reverse and prevent illness.

I have been teaching and practising this new integrated approach to reflexology, combining TCM and diet, for many years. Indeed, my school of reflexology, The International Academy of Reflexology, has campuses around the world and this approach is taught at every one and with great success. Time and time again, people tell me how an understanding of TCM and diet has made them more effective reflexologists.

It is now time to make this knowledge and understanding more wide-ly available and this is what I have set out to achieve with this book: Chapter 1 takes a look at the history of reflexology and how it devel-oped into what we know today; Chapters 2 and 3 introduce the principles of Chinese Medicine and show how they can be applied to reflexology to facilitate more effective healing; Chapter 4 takes a close look at the traditional Chinese systems of the 5 Elements and their 12 meridians from a Western perspective and interprets the traditional characteristics of fire, earth, metal, water and wood for the modern world; Chapter 5 maps the reflexes on the feet; Chapter 6 studies the anatomy, structure and various conditions of the feet; and Chapter 7 shows how to put it all together and give a full reflexology treatment.

It is my hope that this book will make a strong contribution to the understanding of reflexology and that this integrated approach will bring enormous benefits, in terms of health and healing, to practition-ers and patients throughout the world.

I wish you good health and the joy of always feeling fit and full of energy.

Inge Dougans

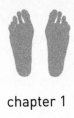

chapter 1

the foundation of modern reflexology

The European Influence

In Europe, a form of reflexology was known and practised as far back as the 14th century. According to Harry Bond Bressler in his book Zone Therapy, pressure therapy was well known in central Europe and was practised by the working classes of those countries as well as by those who catered to the diseases of royalty and the upper classes. Dr Adamus and Dr A'tatis wrote a book on the subject of zone therapy, which was published in 1582; another book on the subject by Dr Ball was published soon after in Leipzig.[1]

The scientific basis of reflex study had its roots in neurological studies conducted in the 1890s by Sir Henry Head of London. In 1898, he discovered zones on the skin which became hypersensitive to pressure when an organ connected by nerves to this skin region was diseased. After years of clinical research, Head established what became known as 'Head's Zones' or 'zones of hyperalgesia'.

Russian work on reflexes began from a psychological point of view. The founder of Russian physiology, Ivan Sechenov (who discovered the cerebral inhibition of spinal reflexes), published a paper in 1870 titled

'Who Must Investigate the Problems of Psychology and How?' Psychologists under Vladimir Bekhterev, founder of Leningrad's Brain Institute, picked up the challenge and studied it through reflexes. At the same time, Ivan Pavlov (1849–1936) read Sechenov's work and acknowledged that his book Reflexes of the Brain was the most important theoretical inspiration for his own work on conditioning. Pavlov took Sechenov's theoretical outline and submitted it to methodical experimental study. Through this, Pavlov developed the theory of conditioned reflexes – namely that there is a simple and direct relationship between a stimulus and a response. Pavlov found that practically any stimulus could act as a conditioning stimulus to produce a conditioned response.[2]

Today the Russians continue to pursue the study of reflexology, both from the physiological and psychological point of view. They have scientifically tested the effect of reflex therapy on patients with a variety of problems and have found reflexology to be an effective complement to traditional medicine.[3]

At the same time, the Germans were also looking into the treatment of disease by massage. In the late 1890s and early 1900s, massage techniques developed in Germany became known as 'reflex massage'. This was the first time that the benefits of massage techniques were credited to reflex actions.

It is possible that Dr Alfons Cornelius was the first to apply massage to 'reflex zones'. The story goes that in 1893 Cornelius suffered from an infection and in the course of his convalescence he received a daily massage. While at the spa he noticed how effective the massages of one particular medical officer were. This man worked longer on areas he found to be painful. This concept inspired Cornelius. After examining himself, Cornelius instructed his masseur to work only on the painful areas. His pain quickly disappeared and in four weeks he recovered completely. This led him to pursue the use of pressure in his own medical practice. He published his manuscript Druckpunkte (or 'Pressure

Points, The Origin and Significance') in 1902.⁴ Europeans went on to expand on the existing research but credit for putting modern reflexology on the map must go to the Americans.

The American Influence

Dr William Fitzgerald, commonly held as the founder of zone therapy, was born in Connecticut, USA, in 1872. He graduated in medicine from the University of Vermont in 1895 and practised in hospitals in Vienna and London. In Vienna, he came into contact with the work of Dr H Bressler, who had been investigating the possibility of treating organs with pressure points. Fitzgerald continued his research while Head Physician at the Hospital for Diseases of the Ear, Nose and Throat in Hartford, Connecticut, testing out many of his theories on his patients. Through knowledge he gained in Europe and his own research, Fitzgerald found that if pressure was applied to the fingers, it would create a local anaesthetic effect on the hand, arm and shoulder, right up to the jaw, face, ear and nose. He applied pressure using tight bands of elastic on the middle section of each finger or small clamps placed on the fingertips. He was able to carry out minor surgical operations using this pressure technique.⁵

Dr Fitzgerald divided the body into zones, which he used for his anaesthetic effect. By exerting pressure on a specific part of the body he learned to predict which other parts of the body would be affected. Fitzgerald established 10 equal longitudinal zones running the length of the body from the top of the head to the tips of the toes. The number 10 corresponds to the fingers and toes and therefore provides a simple numbering system. Each finger and toe falls into one zone. Imagine a line drawn through the centre of the body with 5 zones on either side of this line. The thumb and big toe fall into zone 1 and the small finger and toe both fall into zone 5. The zones are of equal width and extend right through the body from front to back. The theory is that parts of

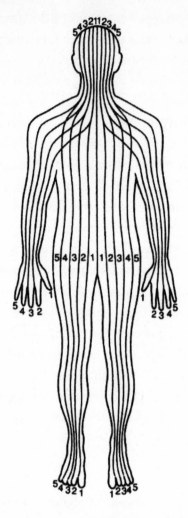

Fig. 1 The Zones

the body found within a certain zone are linked with one another by the energy flow within the zone and can therefore affect one another.

In his book Zone Therapy, Fitzgerald describes how he came upon the concept of zone therapy:

> *'I accidentally discovered that pressure with a cotton-tipped probe on the mucocutaneous margin (where the skin joins the mucous*

membrane) of the nose gave an anaesthetic result as though a cocaine solution had been applied. I further found that there were many spots in the nose, mouth, throat, and on both surfaces of the tongue which, when pressed firmly, deadened definite areas of sensation. Also, those pressures exerted over any body eminence, on the hands, feet, or over the joints, produced the same characteristic results in pain relief. I found also that when pain was relieved, the condition that produced the pain was most generally relieved. This led to my "mapping out" these various areas and their associated connections, and also to noting the conditions influenced through them. This science I have named zone therapy.[6]

Fitzgerald and his colleague Dr Edwin Bowers were so enthusiastic about their discoveries that they developed a unique method for convincing their colleagues about the validity of zone theory. They would apply pressure to the sceptic's hand then stick a pin in the area of the face anaesthetized by the pressure. Such dramatic proof made believers of those who witnessed it. In 1915, Bowers wrote the article that first publicly described this treatment and called it 'zone therapy'. Published in Everybody's Magazine, it was entitled 'To Stop That Toothache Squeeze Your Toe!'[7]

The article elicited much interest and controversy, and Fitzgerald was often called upon to prove publicly the validity of his theories. One such incident was reported in a newspaper on April 29, 1934, under the headline 'Mystery of Zone Therapy Explained'. The article tells of a dinner party at which one of the guests was Fitzgerald and another was a well-known concert singer who had announced that the upper register tones of her voice had gone flat. The article noted that throat specialists had been unable to discover the cause of this affliction. Dr Fitzgerald, according to the article, asked to examine the fingers and toes of the singer. After his examination, he told her that the cause of the loss of her upper tones was a callus on her right big toe. After applying pressure to the corresponding part in the same zone for a few minutes, the patient remarked that the pain in her toe had disappeared. Then, to quote from the article: 'The doctor asked her to try the tone of the upper register. Miraculously, it would seem to us, the singer reached two tones higher than she had ever done before.'[8]

In 1911, the combined work of Dr Fitzgerald and Dr Bowers was published in Zone Therapy. Diagrams of the zones of the feet and the corresponding division of the 10 zones of the body appeared in the first edition of this book. But Fitzgerald did not single out the reflex zones of the feet, so crucial to modern reflexology, for any special attention.

While the medical profession did not receive Fitzgerald and his theories enthusiastically, one physician did believe in his work – Dr Joseph Shelby Riley. Fitzgerald taught zone therapy to Riley and Riley's wife Elizabeth, and they used the method in their medical practice for many years. Riley refined the techniques and made the first detailed diagrams and drawings of the reflex points located in the feet. He added to Fitzgerald's longitudinal zones his discovery of eight horizontal divisions, which also govern the body. His first book, Zone Therapy Simplified, was published in 1919. He went on to write four books in which large portions were devoted to zone therapy.[9]

Fitzgerald, Bower and Riley developed and refined the theory to zone therapy, but it was Riley's assistant Eunice Ingham who probably made the greatest contribution to the establishment of modern reflexology. It was through her untiring research and dedication that reflexology finally came into its own. She separated the work on the reflexes of the feet from zone therapy in general.

Eunice Ingham (1889–1974) should be known as the Mother of Modern Reflexology. She used zone therapy in her work but felt that the feet should be specific targets for therapy because of their highly sensitive nature. She charted the feet in relation to the zones and their effects on the rest of the anatomy until she had drawn up on the feet themselves a 'map' of the entire body. So successful was her work that she is now recognized as the founder of foot reflexology.

Eunice Ingham took her work to the public and the non-medical community because she realized that lay people could learn the proper reflexology techniques to help themselves, their families and friends. She was called on to speak at conventions and shared her knowledge with chiropodists, massage practitioners, physiotherapists, naturopaths and osteopaths. She travelled throughout America for over 30 years as she taught her method through books, charts and seminars to thousands of people in and out of the medical profession. She wrote two books, Stories the Feet Can Tell (1938) and Stories the Feet Have Told (1963). Today her legacy continues under the direction of her nephew Dwight Byers.[10]

The Chinese Connection

To date, most reflexologists have worked with the theory of energy zones described by Dr Fitzgerald. Although this theory has stood reflexology in good stead and contributed greatly to the development of the modern therapy, I do not adhere to it myself. I believe the effects elicited by massaging the feet or hands are largely the result of stimulating the six meridians that run through the feet, as well as the six meridians in the hands. Fitzgerald recognized an energetic connection between the feet and hands with other parts of the body, and without his pioneering work reflexology would not be where it is today. But as the Eastern concept of the meridian system was unknown in the West at the time of his research, the connection with the meridians was not recognized. I, however, am convinced that the energy channels linking the feet and hands to other organs and body parts are the meridians described in Chinese medicine.

Zone theory is considered the basis of modern foot reflexology and most reflexologists use zone theory as a useful adjunct to their work. However, the time has come to take foot reflexology further and expand on existing knowledge by combining it with the ancient Chinese system of meridian therapy. Many believe foot reflexology had its origins in China and developed around the same time as acupuncture. Despite the fact that no definite links can be made, a combination of what is now regarded as primarily a Western development with an ancient Eastern treatment can only be beneficial.

There can be little doubt that a strong link exists between reflexology and acupuncture. They are certainly based on similar ideas. Both are considered meridian therapies as they propose that energy links the hands and feet to various body parts. This enables the whole body to be treated by working on the reflex areas. Acupuncture went from strength to strength in the East but reflexology was, for some reason, lost and forgotten until its recent re-emergence in the West.

The Chinese had divided the body into longitudinal meridians by approximately 2500 BC, whereas the similar idea of zones came to Western awareness as late as the 1900s. Acupuncture, despite its popularity in the East, was an unknown art in the West until 1883, when Dutch physician Ten Thyne wrote a treatise on the subject.

According to acupuncture, the body has 12 pairs of meridians, as well as 2 special meridians known as vessels. Together these constitute the body's energy system, which works to maintain the health of the organism. These meridians are pathways through which the energy of the universe circulates throughout the body organs and keeps the universe and the body in harmony. The acupuncturist believes that illness or pain manifest when the pathways become blocked, disrupting the energy flow and breaking the body's harmony. In acupuncture, the Chinese developed the use of needles to unblock these pathways. In shiatsu, the Japanese use direct thumb and finger pressure on acupuncture meridi-

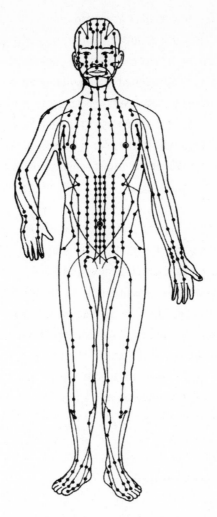

Fig. 2 The meridians

an points to achieve similar results.[11] Reflexologists also work on acupuncture and acupressure points but only those found in the feet and hands. Through increased awareness of meridians, reflexology can be practised more effectively, as meridians provide profound insight into the disease pathway, and are therefore a most useful assessment tool.

The Chinese were undoubtedly aware of the importance of the feet in treating disease. In AD 1017, Dr Wang Wei had a human figure cast in bronze on which were marked those points on the body important for acupuncture. Practitioners put this knowledge into practice in treating the sick, by positioning the needles in the appropriate areas of the body and then applying deep pressure therapy on the soles of the inside and outside edges of both feet. They then applied a concentrated pressure on the big toe. The reason they used the feet in conjunction with the acupuncture needles was to channel extra energy through the body. Dr Wei said that the feet were the most sensitive part of all and contained great energizing areas.[12]

It is not my purpose here to prove that reflexology is directly related to the meridians. The object is to illustrate that a combination of knowledge – modern reflexology techniques and the Eastern meridian system – can be of enormous benefit both to patient and practitioner. As acupuncture and reflexology are concerned with balancing energy flow in order to stimulate the body's own healing potential and restore the state of health, and both are concerned with treating illness in a holistic manner, it seems logical to combine reflexology with meridian therapy in order to provide a more comprehensive and effective treatment programme.

Zones versus Meridians

I am unable to agree with the majority of reflexologists who accept the concept of body congestions being reflected in the longitudinal zones described by Fitzgerald, and am unaware of any definite proof supporting zone theory. I believe reflexology originally developed in conjunction with acupuncture. The reason for massaging the foot was primarily to stimulate the six main meridians that run through the feet. During the course of history, the relationship between these two practices was somehow lost and forgotten. When reflexology re-emerged in the West, researchers and practitioners came to the conclusion that stimulating the feet caused a reaction in the body, but were not sure how this was actuated. As the Eastern meridian knowledge had not at that stage arrived in the West, the relationship with the meridians was not realized, so zone theory was born.

In fact, there are parallels between the meridians and zones. Take, for example, the relationship between the eyes and the kidneys. In zone theory, problems with the eyes can be related to kidney disorders as they both fall into zone 2. This relationship also occurs in the meridians. The bladder meridian begins at the eyes, as does the stomach meridian. The stomach meridian penetrates the kidneys and imbalances may manifest as dark shadows or puffiness under the eyes. Orthodox medicine, too, accepts these signs as being indicative of kidney disorders. The stomach meridian ends in the second toe, with an internal branch of the same meridian in the third toe. Here we have the connection with the toes –the second and third toes represent the eye reflexes and the stomach meridian.

Meridians and Reflexology

The concept of energy channels is the central point around which the practices of reflexology and acupuncture are based. Both function on the premise that vital energy is channelled through the body along specific pathways. In acupuncture, these energy lines are the meridians. In reflexology, as has been perceived to date, the energy channels are those of the zones popularized by Dr W Fitzgerald.

Both practices assert that disease is caused by blockages in energy channels. The acupuncture points, situated all over the body, are usually stimulated or sedated with needles. Reflexology concentrates mainly on the feet, but can also work on the hands, ears or other parts of the body, stimulating with specific finger pressure techniques the reflex areas as well as the sections of meridians situated here.

The six main meridians – those that penetrate the major body organs – are represented in the feet, specifically in the toes. Thus stimulation of the feet helps clear congestions in the meridians. Meridian theory assumes that a disorder within a meridian generates derangement in the pathway and creates disharmony along that meridian, or that such derangement is a result of a disharmony of the meridian's connecting organ. Knowledge of meridians can help reflexologists to understand the disease pathway more comprehensively. A basic knowledge of meridians can be of enormous benefit in pinpointing problem areas. If, for example, pain or irritation does not improve satisfactorily through treatment of the reflex area, one should observe the meridian, which traverses the part of the body in question, and treat the reflex area of the organ related to that particular meridian.

The meridians can be used simply and effectively for a better under-standing of conditions. Take, for example, patients with arthritis in the little finger, tennis elbow, fibrositis in the shoulder blade, swollen lymph glands of the throat, facial nerve disorders or ear disorders such as tin-nitus. One need simply look at the small intestine meridian – this starts in the little finger, ends just in front of the ear and passes the locations of all the above disorders. Could this mean that the small intestine dis-order could aggravate or even cause these problems? Clinical results of balancing the meridians indicate this.

If a patient is suffering from pain in the right knee, question exactly where the pain is situated – on the front, back, medial or lateral section of the knee. If the pain is on the lateral side, it will fall into the gall blad-der meridian. The gall bladder reflex should then be assessed, and will usually be found to be sensitive. Although the organ itself may not be diseased, the congestion on the meridian is causing pain and discomfort.

It is important to distinguish between 'organ conditions' and 'energy conditions'. An 'organ condition' is evident when an organ is not func-tioning properly. This could manifest as digestive or respiratory

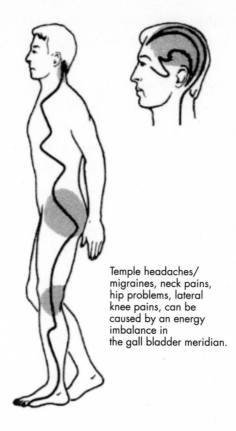

Temple headaches/
migraines, neck pains,
hip problems, lateral
knee pains, can be
caused by an energy
imbalance in
the gall bladder meridian.

Fig. 3a Energy congestions – gall bladder meridian

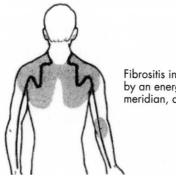

Fibrositis in the shoulder or acne are usually caused
by an energy imbalance in the small intestine
meridian, as is tennis/golfer's elbow

Fig. 3b Energy congestions – small intestine meridian

problems, hormonal disturbances and the like. Energy conditions – for instance, headaches, sciatica, facial nerve disorders and hip pains – are more difficult to define. These conditions are often found along a meridian pathway, and the related organ reflex will usually be sensitive. This does not necessarily indicate an organ disorder. Energy conditions are usually forerunners of more serious problems, and if they are not treated early on, they can eventually influence the related organ and result in a chronic problem. Pains in the fingers and toes often indicate which meridian is congested. For example, pains in the index finger refer to the large intestine meridian, while pains in the big toe could refer to either the liver or spleen/pancreas meridians.

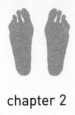

chapter 2

the principles of chinese medicine

'The doctor of the future will give no medicine, but will interest his patients in the care of the human frame, in diet, and in the causes of disease.'

THOMAS EDISON

The main principle of Chinese medicine is based on the saying 'prevention is better than cure', that is, preserving health is preferable to having to treat disease. Disease attacks the body when it is vulnerable. It is the aim of Chinese medicine to build strength by cultivating Chi in order for the body to withstand disease, prevent disease from becoming acute, and protect human life and the conditions that optimize its functioning. The Nei Ching states:

'Maintaining order rather than correcting disorder is the ultimate principle of wisdom. To cure disease after it has appeared is like digging a well when one already feels thirsty, or forging weapons after war has already begun.'

It is interesting to note that Chinese physicians of old were paid when the patient was well, but received no payment when the patient developed any form of disease. To quote the Nei Ching:

> 'The ancient sage did not treat those who were already ill; they
> instructed those who were not ill.'

and

> 'The superior physician helps before the early budding of disease.
> The inferior physician begins to help when the disease has already
> developed; he helps when destruction has already set in. And since
> his help comes when disease has already developed, it is said of
> him that he is ignorant.'

The Nei Ching is widely referred to as the bible of Chinese medicine. The Huang-di Nei-Ching or the Yellow Emperor's Classic of Internal Medicine, the source of all Chinese medical theory, is considered the equivalent of the Corpus Hippocraticum, a group of some 70 texts, compiled by Hippocrates and his followers around 400 BC, that formed the basis for Western medicine. It is the oldest of the Chinese medical texts, dating back about 4,500 years. The Classic of Internal Medicine was believed to have been written by the Yellow Emperor Huang To (2697–96 BC), who reigned in China in about 2600 BC. The book describes conversations between the Yellow Emperor and his royal physician, Chi Po. Given the complexity of the Chinese language, translation of this work has been difficult. The quotations used in this book are derived mainly from the 1972 edition of the translation by Dr Ilza Veith of California University.

Everything is Interconnected – the Web that is Nature

The Chinese medicine viewpoint is based on the systemic approach of the Western world: Human beings are a microcosm within a macrocosm. The Milky Way is a single constellation of stars within the whole universe. Earth is a single planet within the Milky Way. Human beings are only one sub-system within the super-system Earth. The individual organs inside the human body are all smaller sub-systems within the super-system of the human being. All these living systems have an interdependent relationship between them. A change in only one of these systems will have an effect on all the other systems. Chief Seattle placed this interdependent relationship in perspective in 1854 when he said:

> 'This we know – the earth does not belong to man, man belongs to the earth. All things are connected like the blood that unites one family. Whatever befalls the earth befalls the sons of the earth. Man did not weave the web of life; he is merely a strand of it. Whatever he does to the web, he does to himself.'[1]

Living systems are not static. According to the laws of physics, the universe is in constant process, therefore for every action there is an equal and opposite reaction. The same forces or energies of nature that motivate the planets to orbit around Earth and the trees to produce new leaves during spring, motivate human beings to laugh, cry, behave and their organs to function.[2] The balance between all these systems determines our health and hence our quality of life. In nature, imbalances cause forest fires, hurricanes, floods and earthquakes. In the human body, imbalances cause all types of illnesses such as fevers, indigestion, high blood pressure and headaches.

The Tao – the Web

According to Chinese medicine, everything that is and everything that isn't starts with Tao (pronounced dow). What is the Tao? Directly translated, Tao means 'Way'. Tao cannot be defined precisely. It is not tangible and cannot be seen. It is only visible through its various manifestations and is experienced by practising its principles.[3] Tao can also be translated as 'the law of the universe'. It is the dependence of all 'things' on 'no-things' as illustrated by Lao Tze:

> 'We put thirty spokes together and call it a wheel; but it is on the
> space where there is nothing that the usefulness of the wheel
> depends. We turn clay to make a vessel; but it is on the space
> where there is nothing that the usefulness of the vessel depends.'[4]

Tao is 'the root from which all branches grow', 'the source of all substance, energy, awareness.' It is 'a continuum without boundaries in
time and space.'[5] Tao is not a religion; it is a way of life. For years, traditional Eastern philosophy has held, but Western science has confirmed
only recently, that 'matter is nothing more nor less than condensed,
highly organized energy.' Although this is considered to be a scientific
fact, it had not been applied to any medical philosophies of the Western world.[6]

Chi – the Individual Strand of the Web

Chinese philosophy refers to this 'organized energy' as Chi (or Qi, pronounced chee), which originates from and is motivated by Tao. It is the
life force in all its manifestations, such as emotions, tissue, blood,
organs, plants, flowers and animals.[7] Chi flows from the environment
into the human body through low-resistance energy points on the skin,
also known as acupuncture points. These points have electrical properties that differ from the electrical measurements of the surrounding
skin. The sensitivity of these points is determined by the emotional and
physiological changes within the body. Chi flows throughout the
human body in pathways called meridians.

Although it is difficult to measure Chi, indirect evidence of electromagnetic energy circuits involving the meridians and acupuncture points
exists.[8] Chi goes beyond the life-giving energy the human body receives
from ingesting food and breathing air. Chi gives us the inborn urge to
breathe, it 'tells' our hair to grow and our cells to replicate – it is 'the
inner knowing.' It is 'the substance and the activity'; it is each cell and

the activities of each cell in the human body.[9] Once inside the body, Chi provides life energy to all the body organs and body cells through the 12 pairs of meridians. When these meridians allow unobstructed flow of Chi throughout the body, the body is balanced and healthy. But if the Chi is obstructed by congestion, the balance of the body is disturbed and disease will result.

Chi is considered to be 'the root of life', the vital energy within the body that nourishes body and mind.[10] A healthy diet, exercise, healthy breathing, good posture and limited stress will maximize Chi and ensure a healthy individual. A poor diet, lack of exercise, poor breathing and posture, and high levels of stress will deplete Chi, causing imbalances within the system, resulting in disease.

Everyone is born with Chi, and it remains with us until we die. The maintenance of health is dependent on this energy flowing freely throughout the body to animate all the body structure. Chi is constantly depleted through the pressures of daily living and must be correctly cultivated and maintained for healthy functioning.

Two types of Chi are distinguished based on its origin: ancestral Chi/prenatal Chi is inherited from our parents and acquired Chi/postnatal Chi is obtained from the food we eat, the water we drink and the air we breathe.[11] Prenatal Chi is obtained from two sources, the prenatal jing/essence stored in the kidneys (yuan-chi); and from the environment entering the body through the top of the head, the skin and eyes (tien).[12]

Chi is the substance, as well as the physiological functions of the organs, consequently it is in constant motion – 'the activity of life'.[13] It resides in the chest and is associated with breathing, blood, circulation, the heart and lungs. Chi and blood are interdependent – Chi gives blood energy and direction, without Chi blood will stagnate; blood nourishes Chi and gives it form:[14] '... energy leads blood, which means that blood flows wherever energy goes.'[15]

Although Chi cannot be seen, it is believed to have been measured through sensitive electromagnetic machines, and is said to have been photographed by infrared sensitive film. So many scientists in China are now concentrating their research on Chi that a special branch of science has developed called Chi-conology.[16] This research is being conducted with the assistance of practitioners of Qi Gong (or Chi Kung) – an ancient practice that involves controlling the movement of Chi around the body. Qi Gong practitioners can apparently concentrate Chi and expel it out of their bodies, and are reputed to be healthy, strong and less susceptible to disease.

A Question of Energy

As the concept of energy in healing is an important facet of this book, a short introduction is necessary to illustrate how energy is the core which links all living things in the universe.

All matter is made up of energy. The holistic health philosophy considers the human body a dynamic energy system in a constant state of change. We are all an expression of energy and this energy permeates all living organisms. Because we cannot perceive energy with the naked eye, we find it difficult to comprehend. This does not mean it does not exist.

In Chinese and Ayurvedic medicine, health is seen as the fluent and harmonious movement of energies at subtle levels. In the East, these energies have a number of names. The Indian yogis call it prana; to the Tibetan lamas it is lung-gom. It is known as sakia-tundra or ki to the Japanese Shinto, and the Chinese call it Chi. In the West, it is loosely translated as 'vital energy', 'vital force' or 'life force'.

Vital energy represents a form of electricity. This does not mean it is electricity, but its behaviour, responses and reactions indicate that many of the laws applying to electricity also apply to vital energy. Every life function depends on this energy. According to Far Eastern tradition, it circulates in the viscera, the flesh and ultimately permeates every living cell and tissue. This energy is considered as having clearly distinct and established pathways, definite direction of flow, and characteristic behaviour as well defined as any other circulation such as blood and the vascular system.[17]

A great deal of research into Chi and meridians has been conducted in the last few decades, but access to this research is limited for Westerners, as it is published in Chinese. Chinese scientists are thought to be piecing together the fundamental characteristics of life energy. So far, they know it has four characteristics: electric, magnetic, infrared and infrasonic. Says Dr Joshua Le, consultant to the British College of Acupuncture in London: 'Many scientists now believe the electromagnetic recordings of Chi have proved its existence. Everyone has Chi, so it should be acknowledged by everyone, even GPs in the Western world. It's as real as any blood vessels. The significance of this acceptance in medicine worldwide could be tremendous.'[18]

In physical terms, man can be reduced to a collection of electromagnetic fields. What we perceive as solid tissue is actually a mass of cells made up of chemical substances, which are themselves collections of atoms. Every atom carries an electrical charge. An atom consists of protons (positively charged), neutrons (no charge) and electrons (negatively charged). Electrons, being more easily dislodged from atoms than protons, are the main carriers of electrical charge.[19] Thus, at the atomic level, the body is a mass of energy fields, all influencing each other.

The first 'modern' scientific evidence of energy and the human body came from Dr Harold Saxton Burr, Professor of Anatomy at Yale in the 1930s. He was convinced of the existence of 'animal electricity' and developed apparatus to measure electrical potential even in very small organisms. He showed that man, plants and animals are surrounded by a life-field (L-field). Each produces an electrical field that can be measured some distance away from the body and which mirrors – and could possibly even control – changes in that body. 'Animals and plants', said Burr, 'are essentially electric and show a change in voltage gradient associated with fundamental biological activity.'

Burr, the editor of the Yale Journal of Biology and Medicine, published 28 papers outlining the bioelectric nature of menstruation, ovulation, sleep, growth, healing and disease. With his colleagues, he observed that changes in life-fields indicated changes taking place in the organisms producing these fields and he used these to chart the course of health, predict illness, follow the progress of healing in a wound, pinpoint movement of ovulation, diagnose psychic trauma and measure the depth of hypnosis. This energy field or 'aura' can be perceived by 'sensitive' people, and has been 'proven' to exist by Kirlian photography – a technique that photographs the aura.

Another Western physician who made an invaluable contribution to the use of electrical energy in healing is Dr Robert O Becker. An orthopaedic surgeon, he was interested in the possibility of electric current regenerating broken bones. After many experiments on salamanders and frogs to examine electric currents at the site of injury, Becker proved the efficacy of his theory. Now it is possible for patients to have small hearing-aid batteries that produce a sustained negative charge implanted close to severe fractures that are reluctant to heal – with dramatic results. He was also interested in electricity as a factor in the overall control of cell differentiation and growth and he demonstrated that the right kind of current could inhibit infection, relieve pain, halt osteomyelitis, restore muscle control, repair intestinal ruptures, close holes in the heart, regenerate nerve cords and replace lost sections of the brain.[20]

Further research conducted by Dr Bjorn Nordenstrom was revealed in the American magazine Discover. The headline read:

'Electric Man. Dr Bjorn Nordenstrom claims to have found in the human body a heretofore unknown universe of electrical activity that's the very foundation of the healing process and is as critical to well-being as the flow of blood. If he's right, he has made the most profound biochemical discovery of the century.'

Inside, a 13-page article detailed Nordenstrom's discovery of electrical polarities in the bloodstream and how he is manipulating the natural electrical circuits he has found to disperse tumours.[21]

Dr Randolph Stone, who died in 1981 in India at the age of 91, combined Eastern and Western understanding to develop Polarity Therapy. A qualified osteopath and chiropractor, he came to define techniques for balancing the energy flow in human beings through his knowledge of Eastern wisdom, his understanding of the inner structure of the universe and of the gunas, the three fundamental attributes of Ayurvedic medicine, described in Hindu literature. He developed, practised and taught Polarity Therapy in California and India with great success.[22]

The West has finally discovered what the East has acknowledged for thousands of years – that a kind of electrical energy forms the basis of all life. More people are beginning to accept that the physical world is part of a much larger whole – a whole that, unfortunately, most of us cannot physically perceive. We pick up only a tiny fraction of what is really going on around us, because our concepts of life are limited by our five physical senses.

To quote Lyall Watson's book Supernature II:

'Earth and everything in it is under constant bombardment. We are battered by a ceaseless barrage of more than a hundred million impulses every second, a confusing avalanche of raw knowledge with which we cannot hope to deal.

'The flood ranges from highly energetic cosmic rays, whose origin remains mysterious, but which at all latitudes have the intriguing property of coming rushing in largely from the West; through shortwave gamma and X-radiation, which passes with relative ease through our bodies; to ultraviolet and infra-red light waves that leave us with Vitamin D and radiant heat; and a wide band of radio frequencies that bring us sound broadcasting, television, radar and a scattering of information about distant galaxies in collision.

'Most of this news is irrelevant. It contributes nothing to an organism battling for survival on a much more limited field. To prevent being overwhelmed by the flood, we have evolved barriers, which filter out the stuff we don't need.

'So, from all the pyrotechnics of electromagnetism our senses select just that narrow band of radiation that represents the visible spectrum –those wavelengths which lie between 375 and 775 billionths of a metre. We look on the world through a tiny slit, and this narrow window on reality is even further restricted by the censorship-taking place between the eye and the brain.'[23]

The human ear responds to sounds within a frequency range of approximately 30–16,000 cycles per second. Human vision responds to wavelengths from 380 to 760 mill microns. Of approximately 50 octaves of electromagnetic radiations, our eyes pick up less than 1.

From the barrage of electromagnetic waves in the environment, living organisms select only those necessary for their survival. Although our brains are not geared to pick up TV waves, radio waves and ultrasonic frequencies, we do not doubt their existence, so it is clearly unwise to doubt the existence of electrical energy in the body merely because we cannot see it.

All life on Earth is intricately interwoven with the natural rhythms and laws of the universe. Every organism regulates its metabolic activity in cycles attuned to the fluctuations of the earth, sun and moon. So cosmic forces directly and indirectly have an effect on us humans which is beyond our control. To quote Lyall Watson again:

> 'Our internal clocks are clearly tied to the rhythms provided by the planet and its nearest neighbours in the solar system. We wake and sleep, sweat and shiver, urinate and breathe in time with cosmic cues that are often so subtle that medical science has had a hard time taking them seriously. But an avalanche of studies in the last (few) decades on insomnia, menstrual irregularity and stress in those suffering from cyclic disturbances such as jet lag has turned the tide. It is now more widely accepted that functional integrity, the basic processes of growth and control, and the efficient working of the central nervous system are all maintained to a very large extent by our electromagnetic environment.'[24]

This brief synopsis barely begins to encompass the vastness and multiplicity of phenomena occurring around us all the time, but it is intended to emphasize the importance of the interconnectedness of all things and how health is dependent on vital electrical forces. The optimum state for each individual is to live in harmony with nature and the surrounding environment. And it is the role of the reflexologist, working in accordance with holistic philosophy, to help people to work towards and achieve this state of balance.

Yin/Yang Theory

Yin and yang is the earliest scientific principle recorded in traditional Chinese medicine. It replaced superstition, as all changes were previously explained in terms of spirits and demons.[25] Yin and yang are the two forces that move the world, two manifestations of being, and two complementary and contrasting energies. For the Chinese, yin and yang do not exist separately – they correspond to the two sides of the same coin; being a single principle they cannot exist in isolation. Day and night are inseparable; one cannot exist without the other. Yin and yang are in a state of continuous movement. Energy is not stagnant – by definition it moves. Pathologies, therefore, are energy blockages caused by excess or deficiency.

Yin and yang are two opposite but complementary and interdependent poles of the energy or Chi generated by Tao.[26] Ilza Veith, in the introduction to her translation of The Yellow Emperor's Classic of Internal Medicine states: '... Yin and Yang were conceived as one entity and that both together were ever-present.' Nature as a whole, including human beings, is composed of these two forces, in other words a yin or yang 'value' can be designated for all phenomena, including cosmic processes. These two opposing energy forces are relative to and interdependent on each other. A yin is only a yin in the presence of a yang and vice versa. Chee Soo illustrates this interdependent relationship between yin and yang with the following metaphor: 'For a cup (yang) is only a cup when you have a void (yin) in the centre.'[27]

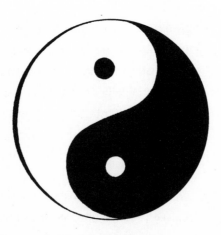

Fig. 1 Yin/yang symbol

In reality, neither of these two forces are absolute – yin has a little piece of yang in it and yang has a little piece of yin in it (previous page). Under certain conditions, yin can become yang and vice versa. This ability to transmute initiates all changes in nature, as a change in one element will affect all other elements, due to their interdependent relationship. Yang is illustrated in traditional Chinese medicine as the 'sunny side of the mountain'. It represents the male principle: active, positive, heat, fire, light, fat, dryness, the sun, it flows upwards and outwards and expands. The 'dark side of the mountain' illustrates yin.[28] It represents the female element: negative, passive, cold, thin, destructive, the moon, the Earth, night, water, dampness, darkness, death, it flows downward and contracts. In order to obtain balance or equilibrium, both of these opposing energy forces must be present: for example, in order to have birth there must be death, to have day there must be night, to have movement there must be stasis.[29]

Note: The fact that yang represents the positive and yin represents the negative does not imply that yang has a positive value and yin has a negative value. It is purely an indication that they are two opposing polarities. No deeper interpretation, meaning or value should be attached than this.

It is said that heaven was created by the accumulation of yang and that Earth was created by the accumulation of yin.[30] Human beings are the result of the interaction between the yang of heaven and the yin of Earth – the 'offspring of their union'.[31] Humans draw energy or Chi from heaven and Earth and transform it into an energy system suitable for the body's organs and their functions.[32] Implicit in this is the fact that human beings are interwoven with nature and cannot be separated from it.

The polarity of yin and yang therefore also applies to humans in terms of the structure and functions of their bodies. It guides the functions of every organ in the body, and organs are paired relative to each other according to the yin/yang principle.[33] Traditional Chinese Medicine (TCM) uses the principle of yin/yang to analyze, diagnose and treat a disease. Yang symptoms, according to TCM, are fever, sweating, constipation, chronic thirst, dry lips and mouth, dark urine, heavy breathing, rapid pulse and irritability. Yin symptoms are loose bowels, lack of thirst, shallow breathing, slow pulse, lethargy, chills, cold hands and feet (circulation).[34] Illness manifests as external symptoms, which is an indication of a yin/yang imbalance inside the body or between the body and its environment.[35] In treatment, TCM aims to correct this imbalance, which will bring natural relief of the symptoms. Western medicine, on the other hand, focuses on relieving the symptoms only, irrespective of its cause.

A healthy body has the ability to adapt rapidly and to alter constantly the proportion of yin to yang (and vice versa). In this way, balance is maintained throughout the body and disease is prevented. A body that lacks the ability to change and adapt will carry an extreme yin or yang polarity. This will cause an imbalance and consequently make the body prone to disease.[36] Beinfield and Korngold describe this state of imbalance and disease thus: 'The man is not sick because he has an illness, but has an illness because he is sick.' Perfect balance between yin and yang within the body and between the body and external environment, implies a healthy body, mind and spirit.

The Theory of the Five Elements

It is said that the theory of the Five Elements or five phases was introduced to Chinese medicine from India. The Five Elements are created due to the interaction between yin and yang, which is why the Five Elements are also considered to be energies. The Five Elements can be viewed as the manifestation and behaviour of Chi within five specific cycles.

In this way, five interdependent, opposing and complementing cycles (energies) of transformation were identified within the yin/yang principle: birth, adulthood, maturity, aging/degeneration and dying. The Taoists gave these cycles names: birth (wood), adulthood (fire), maturity (earth), aging/degeneration (metal) and dying (water).[37] A change in one of the elements will affect all the other elements. The dynamics of the Five Elements describe the process of change within an organism and between an organism and its environment. An ancient Chinese treatise states: 'By the transformation of yang and its union with yin, the Five Elemental Energies of Wood, Fire, Earth, Metal, and Water arise, each with its own specific nature according to its share of yin and yang.'[38]

Wood is associated with active functions and growth, fire includes functions that have reached a maximum state of activity and are about to decline to a resting period, earth represents a neutral state of balance, metal includes functions in a declining state and water reflects those functions that have reached a state of maximum rest preparing to change direction in activity.[39] The Five phases are evident in all aspects of nature: 'All things contain all Five Elemental Energies in various proportions.' The seasons manifest through these five phases: spring (wood), summer (fire), late summer (earth), autumn (metal), winter (water). Because human beings are part of nature, these five energy cycles are applied to the human system, their physical, sensory, perceptual, emotional, intellectual and spiritual life.[40] Ilza Veith writes:

> 'Man who is said to be the product of heaven and earth by the interaction of Yin and Yang also contains, therefore, the Five Elements.'

In this light, Five Element theory was extended to include human behaviour.[41] The relationship between the Five Elements forms the basis for the prevention, assessment and treatment of disease, as it describes the physiology of the human body in relation to its environment. The

Five Elements are interdependent and interaction between these elements happens in two cycles reflecting our yin/yang nature.

A generating cycle/yin cycle

This cycle is also referred to as the 'Mother–Son Law', as each element is the 'mother' of the next element and the 'son' of the previous element. Each element produces the next element and supplies it with energy – wood creates fire, fire creates earth, earth creates metal, metal creates water, water creates wood. In the context of the natural world, the following cycle occurs: wood burns creating fire, fire produces ashes creating earth, earth holds within it different minerals represented by metal, metal is a mineral of the earth and in liquid form it is similar to water, water gives life to wood which is represented by the trees and plants; the cycle then starts again.[42] It is important to note that no single element has more value than another. Each element and the functions it performs are important, as they are all interdependent.

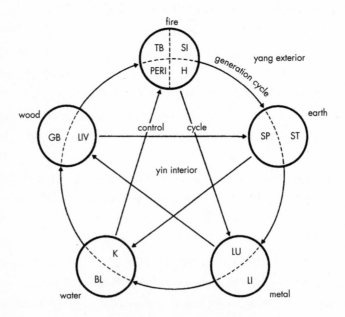

Fig. 2 Generating/control cycle

A control cycle/yang cycle

Each element exerts a type of control over another in order to maintain balance throughout the system. If one element becomes too strong it will 'attack' and 'injure' another element. By the same token, if an element becomes too weak it will be 'attacked' and 'injured' by another element. This will result in an unbalanced system. In nature, this control cycle is evident in the way that wood controls earth by means of roots keeping the soil in place and preventing erosion; on the other hand, roots can also uproot earth and deplete it by drawing out nutrients from the earth. Earth exerts control over water by providing boundaries, so preventing flooding; however, earth can also restrict water from flowing freely when it dams or absorbs water. Water controls fire by preventing it from blazing and getting out of control, yet water can also extinguish fire. Fire controls metal by allowing it to be flexible and take on different forms by softening or melting it. Metal controls wood by cutting or chopping it down, preventing it from becoming overgrown and allowing space for other living organisms; but metal can also destroy wood completely by cutting too much down.[43]

- Wood generates fire by controlling earth;
- Fire generates earth by controlling metal;
- Earth promotes metal by controlling water;
- Metal promotes water by controlling wood;
- Water promotes wood by controlling fire.

The following example illustrates the interaction between the Five Elements from a Western medicine and a traditional Chinese medicine point of view. During congestive heart (fire) failure, changes in the lungs (metal) occur due to the fact that the blood can no longer flow to and from the lungs in order to excrete carbon dioxide and absorb oxygen. The affected lungs will subsequently cause cellular dysfunctions in the liver (wood). The congestive heart failure also causes pressure and congestion in the liver due to blood accumulating in the veins feeding the liver. The malfunctioning of the liver (wood) causes malfunctions in the spleen (earth).[44]

The yin and yang cycles operate simultaneously, creating a feedback system, in order to bring about and maintain balance in nature and throughout the human body.[45]

Every person has a natural and spontaneous affinity towards one of the elements. All Five Elements exert an influence in one's life, but one will be manifest stronger than the others. Together, the Five Elements have a direct influence on a person's personality, emotions, spiritual needs and predisposition to physical weaknesses. The two opposing but comple-mentary cycles containing the Five Elements, being yin and yang, operate simultaneously in order to achieve balance in nature, as well as through-out the human body. Balance will result in good health, while imbalances between the elements and its two cycles will result in disease.[46]

A detailed analysis on each of the Five Elements is provided later in this book (see pages 69–174). It is first necessary to understand a few fur-ther theories underlying TCM, as these theories will be integrated within the analysis of the individual elements.

Examination and Diagnosis

During examination, information is gathered in order to identify the symptoms, which will indicate any underlying imbalances. Analysis classifies these imbalances, and a decision is made as to how they will be treated and the balance restored.

The information obtained from the examination is integrated and organized, utilizing the principles of TCM to identify a specific group of symptoms. These groups of symptoms are referred to as symptom-com-plexes.[47] A symptom-complex goes beyond a symptom. It is a summary of the functioning of the body at a specific phase or stage of the disease. It includes the symptoms manifested and connects these symptoms to imbalances in the body. The cause of the imbalances, location and nature of the disease are then identified. A decision is made based on these findings with regards to the treatment required.[48] The aim of the treatment is to regulate the relationship between the factors of the symptom-complex by applying the yin/yang theory, restoring balance to the meridians and consequently the whole body.

The patient is always examined and assessed from the following perspective: the body functions as a whole, all body parts are interdependent, and the body and its environment are interdependent. Ohashi illustrates this interdependency when he says:

> 'In Oriental diagnosis, we see the body as an orchestra whose music is the soul. Remove any instrument, or change the way it is played, and you alter the music entirely. To bring out the full breadth of the spirit, you must finely tune each organ as if it were an instrument. It must function optimally, as if a virtuoso was playing it. Yet you must never forget that each organ must blend harmoniously with the rest of the body – all the other pieces of the orchestra – to bring forth the most complete and beautiful being, which is you. The Oriental healer, therefore, is like the conductor of an orchestra. He or she hears the instruments that are playing out of tune and adjusts them to bring each into harmony with the rest of the orchestra.'[49]

The Theory of the Causes of Disease

The causes of disease are inherent to the theory of the Five Elements. As we have seen, the Five Elements are manifestations of the vital life-giving energy or Chi. Balance between the Five Elements, and therefore the flow of Chi, will promote and maintain longevity and good health.

Imbalances in any of the Five Elements, implies an imbalance in the flow of Chi, which will result in disease. According to TCM, disease derives from one of two causes.

Environmental factors

If the human body lacks the ability to protect itself from harmful external environmental factors, imbalances will occur and disease will result. These factors are related to abnormal climatic conditions. When climatic conditions are in excess or lacking it disturbs the balance between the body and the environment.[50] Chinese medicine refers to these abnormal climatic conditions as 'the five devils'. The five devils are associated with the Five Elements and the major organs inside the human body.

- Wood is related to the climate wind, affecting the gall bladder and liver;
- Fire is associated with the climate heat and affect the heart, small intestines, circulation and triple burner;
- Earth is associated with the climate dampness, affecting the stomach, spleen and pancreas;
- Metal is related to the climate dryness and affect the lungs and large intestine;
- Water is related to a cold climate affecting the bladder and kidneys.

The degree to which each of the climatic conditions will influence the individual is dependent on his/her affinity with each climatic condition and the strength of their Chi to protect the body against these external attacks.

While Western medicine identifies the external factors causing disease as bacteria and viruses, Chinese medicine does not specifically refer to these as external causes of disease. However, they can be accommodated within the Chinese medicine paradigm.[51]

Internal dysfunctions

Internal dysfunctions in the human body are related to extreme, intense emotions. These are referred to as the 'five destructive emotions' and they are associated with the Five Elements and with the major organs of the human body. The Five Elements are related to the five emotions as follows:

- Wood is related to anger, affecting the gall bladder and the liver;
- Fire is related to joy, affecting the heart and small intestines, circulation/pericardium and the triple burner;
- Water is related to fear, affecting the bladder and kidneys;
- Metal is related to grief and worry, affecting the lungs and large intestines;
- Earth is related to sympathy and needs, affecting the stomach, spleen and pancreas.

When one or more of these emotions is experienced in extremity and excess, or when we are unable to express or experience these emotions properly, this causes imbalances in the Chi flowing through the body. These imbalances deplete the body's ability to protect itself against both internal and external attacks on the body and disease will result. Other internal causes of disease include tension, overexertion, dietary maladjustments, excess sexual activity, excess mucus, blood clotting, and heredity dysfunctions.[52]

All these internal and external factors are interdependent and their interaction with each other leads to specific groups of symptoms. These symptoms are manifested physically (external or internal) and emotionally (in terms of behaviour) as described by the dynamics of the Five Elements and are indications of imbalances within one or more of the elements.[53]

Today we are once again beginning to learn what the Chinese knew thousands of years ago, that disease is mostly the result of wrong living – not living in accord with the natural laws of the universe. Ancient Chinese philosophy regarded the human organism as a miniature version of the universe and often referred to man as 'the small world'. Thus, man cannot be divorced from nature as he forms an organic part of it. Nature as macrocosm and man as microcosm obey the same laws. The Nei Ching says:

> 'Those who rebel against the basic rules of the universe sever their own roots and ruin their true selves. Yin and yang, the two principles in nature, and the four seasons are the beginning and the end of everything and they are also the cause of life and death. Those who disobey the laws of the universe will give rise to calamities and visitations, while those who follow the laws of the universe remain free from dangerous illness, and they are the ones who have obtained Tao, the Right Way.'

Meridian Theory

The meridian theory represents the anatomy of the human body according to Chinese medicine. The Nei Ching states:

> 'The Meridians move the Chi and Blood, regulate the Yin and the Yang, moisten the tendons and the Bones, and benefit the joints ... internally the Meridians connect with the Organs and externally with the joints, limbs and the outer surface of the body.'[54]

The meridians are a network of energy channels of which there are 12 major ones (see page 38). Each meridian passing through the one side of the body has a mirror image on the other side of the body, resulting in 12 pairs of meridians. In order to maintain health, the circulatory and nervous system must be able to flow uninterrupted throughout the body; if it is not something is bound to go wrong. The same principle applies to the meridian network. When Chi flows uninterrupted throughout the body via the meridians, good health will be achieved and maintained. The environment (external factors), our thoughts and emotions (internal factors), and what we eat, drink and breathe all affect the flow of Chi in the meridian network, as indicated by the theory of the Five Elements.[55]

The flow of energy or Chi through the meridians happens in specific cycles within a 24-hour period. The energy flows at a maximum level for a period of 2 hours in each meridian and at a minimum level 12 hours later. This implies that a specific meridian and its connecting organ will dominate the body during a specific 2-hour period. If the Chi in this meridian is in shortage and consequently imbalanced, related symptoms will be felt intensely during this time period. (This is discussed in more detail in Chapter 4 under each individual meridian.)

Acupuncture or acupressure points are located along each meridian, which are linked to the structure of the organs. If a meridian is congested, stimulation of these points will allow energy to enter the meridians. Alternatively, if a meridian is overloaded with energy, stimulation of the acupuncture points will release the excess energy.[56] Stimulation of the meridians clears congestions, and restores balance and health within the body, hence improving the flow of Chi.

Western medicine recognizes a nervous system and a circulatory system within the human body, but focuses on the structure and functions of each individual organ. Although, for instance, the circulatory system supplies each organ with the nourishment necessary to allow the functioning of all organs possible, Western medicine does not consider this interrelationship as significant. Western medicine sees the circulatory system as just another organ and analyzes it in terms of its structure and functions separate from all the other organs. In TCM, each individual organ is understood in terms of its functions and its structure.

However, the structure of each organ is not looked at solely in terms of the cells, membranes and mechanisms that go to make it up. Instead, the structure of each organ consists of the organ and the meridian responsible for nourishing that specific organ with live-giving Chi. Included in the structure of each organ is how that organ relates to, influences and is influenced by the other organs and their meridians, as indicated by the theory of the Five Elements.

Although we refer to 12 major meridians, in fact there is only one single meridian running throughout the whole body, as all of these meridians are connected to each other, flowing into one another. They are bilateral (paired), giving 24 separate pathways. Each meridian is connected and related to a specific organ from which it gets its name – in most cases the organs are ones with which we are familiar. In addition, it is connected to a coupled meridian and organ with which it has a specific relationship. The coupled meridians consist of a yin and yang aspect, and come under the dominance of one of the five elements (see table below).

ELEMENT	YANG ORGAN	YIN ORGAN
Wood	Gall bladder	Liver
Fire	Small Intestine/Triple Burner	Heart/Circulation
Earth	Stomach	Spleen/Pancreas
Metal	Large Intestine	Lungs
Water	Bladder	Kidneys

It is difficult to draw a dividing line between the anatomical and physiological concepts of the Nei Ching. The organs are described for their function rather than for their location and structure, and the idea of cosmology (the continuous interaction of yin and yang, the four seasons and the five elements) dominates the theories of structure as well as those of function.

According to the Nei Ching, the body has five 'viscera' and six 'bowels'. The viscera, which are yin, are the heart, spleen, lungs, liver and kidneys. These have the capacity to store but not eliminate. They determine the function of all the other parts of the body, including the bowels, and also of the spiritual resources and emotions. The function of yin organs is to produce, transform, regulate and store the fundamental substances – chi, blood, Jing, shen (spirit) and body fluids. Jing is best translated as 'essence' and is the substance that underlies all organic life. It is the source of organic change and is generally thought of as fluid-like. Jing is supportive and nutritive and is the basis of reproduction and development.

The six bowels are yang organs and have the capacity of elimination but not of storing. These are the gall bladder, stomach, large intestine, small intestine, bladder and the triple burner (triple heater or three burning spaces). The triple burner is not an actual organ, and will be discussed in more depth in the detailed description of the meridians (see chapter 4). The yang organs receive, break down and absorb that part of the food that will be transformed into fundamental substances, and transport and excrete unused portions.

The position of the viscera and bowels is compared to that of various officials in an empire, relating to the 12 main organs and meridians. The 12 officials must always work together for the maintenance of the whole, and never fail to assist one another.

> 'When the monarch is intelligent and enlightened, there is peace and contentment among his subjects; thus they can beget offspring, bring up their children, earn a living, and lead a long and happy life. And because there are no more dangers and perils, the earth is considered glorious and prosperous.'

In addition to the 12 organ meridians, there are also 2 'vessel' meridians termed the 'governing' and 'conception' meridians. They serve as

energy reservoirs for the entire meridian network. The governing meridian (the Du channel) stores energy for and supplies energy to all the
yang meridians within the body. It has its origin in the pelvic cavity.
From there it descends internally, surfacing at the perineum, passing
through the tip of the coccyx. It ascends along the spine, the neck, over
the head, descends along the middle of the forehead and nose, ending
inside the upper gum. A smaller internal branch ascends from the pelvic
cavity, through the buttocks to the kidneys. Another small internal
branch leaves the main meridian at the base of the head and enters the
brain.[57]

The conception meridian (the Ren channel) stores Chi and supplies it to
all the yin meridians. It is called the conception meridian as it is thought
that in women it originates in the uterus and is responsible for the
development of the foetus. This meridian starts in the pelvic cavity,
emerging at the perineum and ascends over the middle of the pubic
area. From there it ascends along the middle of the abdominal area, the
chest and throat to the chin. Here it penetrates and encircles the lips
internally. Two internal branches pass from the lips on either side of the
nose ascending over the cheeks, parallel with the nose ending underneath each eye.[58]

The meridians all have two sections – one section is close to the surface
of the body and the other is internal and deeper inside the body. Each
meridian and its connecting organ can be classified in terms of the
yin/yang principle. Organs that are hollow, most often externally situated within the body cavities and involved in the process of discharging
substances, are considered to be yang organs. These organs are responsible for the reception, transmission and digestion of food and liquids
and the elimination of wastes. Solid organs, positioned more internally
in the body and involved in the absorption, regulation and storing of
various substances are considered to be yin organs. The meridians connecting these organs can be classified as supplying these organs with
either yang or yin Chi. The meridian energy network connects the envi-

ronment surrounding the body to the internal organs. The course of each meridian plays an essential role in the diagnosis and treatment of diseases, as postulated by traditional Chinese medicine.

To recap, reflexology works to help attain and maintain the equilibrium in the Chi by activating the sections of the meridians present on the feet, as well as activating the reflexes of the organs relating to each of the meridians. This is why it is important to incorporate the concept of meridian therapy with the practice of reflexology.

Chinese medicine is essentially holistic. It is based on the idea that disease cannot be isolated from the patient and that no single part can be understood except in its relation to the whole. Nothing is treated symptomatically. According to the Nei Ching:

'Illness is comparable to the root; good medical work is comparable to the topmost branch; if the root is not reached, the evil influences cannot be subjugated.'

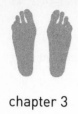

chapter 3

applying a knowledge of the meridians in reflexology

'Tell me and I'll forget. Show me and I may remember but involve me and I'll understand.'

ANCIENT CHINESE PROVERB

As Ted Kaptchuk explains in The Web That Has No Weaver:

'To Western medicine, understanding an illness means uncovering a distinct entity that is separate from the patient's being; to Chinese medicine, understanding means perceiving the relationships between the patient's signs and symptoms ... The Chinese method is thus holistic, based on the idea that no single part can be understood except in its relation to the whole ... If a person has a symptom, Chinese medicine wants to know how the symptom fits into the patient's entire bodily pattern ... Understanding that overall pattern, with the symptom as part of it, is the challenge of Chinese medicine.'

Using needles, cupping or thumb and finger pressure on the acupuncture points to stabilize and harmonize the flow of Chi in the meridians, an important reflexology tool uses the concept of congestions within the meridians as an assessment technique.

As we have seen, congestions result from blockages along the meridians, thus obstructing the flow of vital energy or Chi. Congestion such as sinus problems, tennis elbow, breast lumps, headaches or knee pain, has at its root the same problem. For each organ to maintain a state of perfect health, the Chi must be able to flow freely along the meridians. The meridian system unifies all parts of the body and is essential for the maintenance of harmonious balance.

The atom, the basic form of an element, is composed of a central nucleus formed of protons and neutrons, around which electrons revolve. One of the largest entities we know of is the solar system, which has a similar structure to the atom: the sun the central nucleus with planets revolving around it. A group of atoms makes up a molecule, a group of molecules forms a cell, groups of cells form tissue, a mass of tissue forms an organ, a group of organs forms a system, a number of systems become a person, several persons make up a family, many families form a tribe, a clan or neighbourhood, many neighbourhoods make a town, many towns a province, and so on. Thus, one is in everything and everything is in one. In every part of the body, we find the whole body projected proportionately in an organic, precise, logical way.

If we accept the viewpoint of human beings as multidimensional bodies of energy, it follows that human beings can be affected by energy. We need to understand that energy, the Chi being referred to here is a vibration, and everything on our planet consist of vibrational energy. Reflexology, acupuncture and many other therapies are in basic essence, vibrational therapies.

Vibration is a synonym for frequency – different frequencies of energy reflecting varying rates of vibration. We know that matter and energy are manifestations of the same primary energetic substance of which everything in the universe is composed, including our physical and subtle bodies. The vibratory rate of this universal energy determines the density of its expression or form as matter. Matter, which vibrates at a very slow frequency, is referred to as physical matter. That which vibrates at speeds exceeding the velocity of light is known as subtle matter. In order to therapeutically impact on the system, energy needs to be administered that vibrates at frequencies beyond the physical plane.

Vibrational medicines such as homeopathic tinctures or flower essences are thought to be charged with a particular frequency of subtle energy. These subtle energetic patterns, which are stored within the vibrational essence, may be used to affect human beings at a variety of interactive levels.

> 'The acupuncturists see meridian dysfunction as a precursor of organ pathology. The meridian circuit abnormality reflects an imbalance in the polar energies of the forces of yin and yang. Neither force exists alone, but in relation to the total energetic needs of the organism.'
>
> RICHARD GERBER, VIBRATIONAL MEDICINE

It is at this level that we need to consider the impact of reflexology treatments on the human system. The stimulation of reflexes and meridians we practise generates vibrational waves which, on reaching a target organ or congestion, trigger a chemical reaction in the body; our body reacts to two fundamental stimuli – contraction and expansion – which we can translate into heat-cold stimuli, or yin and yang.

Congestion of the Meridians

Cooking and eating good food are the cornerstones of human civilization, however what we eat has consequences for the amount of Chi we receive to keep the meridians and therefore our body and mind in a healthy state.

As we have seen, subtle energy vibrates at different frequencies – the lower the frequency, the more solid the matter will be. This means that food which is dense is likely to be stagnant and so congest the meridian pathways. For this reason it is important to make sure that what we eat is as pure as possible.

The vibration of our food is increasingly dense as most is man-made with high levels of non-digestible and non-biodegradable chemicals. Hormone expert Dr John Lee made the following comment with regard to xenoestrogens – empty oestrogens that mimic real oestrogens and take the latter's place in the body:

> 'Xenoestrogens from the environment come from pesticide residues, industrial residues and plastics, which contaminate water and get into the food chain. Research has shown that the combination of tiny amounts of these hormone-disrupting chemicals, equivalent to the levels found in human blood, is carcinogenic and triggers breast cells to proliferate.'

These alterations in our food chains are the major underlying cause of many of our most devastating diseases such as cancer, heart disease, obesity, mental imbalances, as well as the many widespread intolerances and allergies. Pure food, naturally grown, such as vegetables, herbs and fruits which have not been genetically modified, treated with hormones, chemically fertilized or cold stored, have a much higher vibration supplying us with a greater level of Chi.

High vibrational food

On the whole, if we buy commercially grown fruits and compare their aroma to that of organically grown equivalent, which have been allowed to ripen naturally on the tree or bush influenced by the sun's rays, a marked difference will be found. A ripe, red sun-grown tomato, picked directly from the garden is deliciously sweet and has a strong pleasant aroma. By comparison, a commercially grown tomato has very little aroma, and the sweetness is almost undetectable. There is a crucial difference between the vibrational patterns of these two tomatoes. The one that has been left to ripen naturally under the sun in healthy soil has the optimum balance between its sodium and potassium, as well as other minerals, thus giving it a high vibrational pattern, as well as being alkaline forming.

The tomato which was commercially grown and picked green, not allowing the sodium and potassium to become balanced by the action of the sun's rays, and which may contain many pollutant chemicals, will have a lower vibrational pattern resulting in a tomato with little or no aroma or sweetness, as well as being acid forming.

Although we may be under the impression that we are eating very healthily when we eat much fruit and vegetables, this may not be the case if they are grown in such a way as to distort the mineral content and therefore the Chi.

This illustrates how important it is not only that we eat healthily from the point of view of food groups, but also from the point of view of vibrational energy – or Chi.

The Thoughts We Think – and the Feelings We Have

As humans we are energy and we are sustained by energy. Our bodies are ever-changing, dynamic fields of energy and not static physical structures. Every part of our body contains information about the whole. We know from quantum physics that at the sub-atomic level, matter and energy are interchangeable. Christine Northrup in Women's Bodies, Women's Wisdom, uses the expression: 'Matter is the densest form of spirit and spirit is the lightest form of matter.'

When you are confronted with or you are the recipient of negative, hurtful or destructive actions, you experience negative thoughts and feelings. If you do not let go of those feelings, they become heavy dense vibrations. And this energy vibration will manifest somewhere, maybe in the subtle body or maybe in the physical body. Furthermore, it will drain the Chi that is otherwise needed for homeostasis. Caroline Myss, in her book Anatomy of the Spirit, brings it together concisely when she says that 'your biography becomes your biology'.

How Much Chi do We Need?

Food labelling on most man-made products indicates the amount of kilojoules or calories they contain, converting them into a measure of energy. In addition, an indication of the content of fat, vitamins, colouring and preservatives using E-numbers gives the consumer an estimated idea of what they are eating. Lifestyle experts have worked out how many kilojoules an average male and female will need in order to stay healthy and active without too much of a weight problem – yet the developed world is becoming obese and lethargic with many diseases relating to a weak immune system.

However, no food labelling gives the Chi content of a product, nor do we know how much Chi we need for our meridians to function optimally, thereby supplying our cells, tissues and organs with the correct amount in order to experience homeostasis.

As an analogy, vital energy may be seen as a form of electricity. This does not mean it is electricity, but that its behaviour, responses and reactions indicate that many of the laws applying to electricity also apply to vital energy – Chi. Every life function depends on this energy. According to Eastern tradition, it circulates in the viscera, the flesh and, ultimately, permeates every cell and tissue.

According to Chinese medicine, the body has 12 pairs of meridians, as well as 2 special meridians. Together these constitute the body's energy system, which works to maintain the health of the human body. The meridians are pathways forming a continuous circuit through which the universal energy – the life force, the Chi – circulates. It circulates through the body organs and keeps the energetic system of the body in harmony. In these terms, the meridians can be thought of as electrical pathways, which can be used as an assessment tool by warning us that there is insufficient energy running through them.

Internal branch congestions versus meridian congestions

Throughout the artwork of the meridians found in this book, you will see dotted and solid lines, representing 'Internal Branches' and 'Meridians'.

When I first wrote The Art of Reflexology in the late 1980s, I came across this division, although scarce information was then available on the subject. Since then, I have since come to appreciate the difference and have added my own interpretation. The 'normal' meridian is illustrated with the solid line and the internal with the dotted line.

To continue the electrical analogy, when we flick a switch in our home, we automatically have electricity supplying us with power; however, we rarely even consider the source. With the meridians, the idea is very similar. The meridians (solid lines) can be compared to outdoor electricity. Each streetlight can be likened to an acupuncture point, which is an amplifier for this electricity. These are needed because without boosters the effect of the electricity would be weakened and eventually lost over the course of the circuit. Our acupuncture points are like these electrical amplifiers; when stimulated they release blockages along the pathways, amplifying the energy and allowing it to flow freely again. This is one way to try and visualize the internal meridian.

The external meridians differ from the internal meridians, as they warn us of potential blackouts in our electricity (Chi) supply, by means of congestions along the pathways. In order that each of the 12 meridians are at their optimum balance, feeding every cell, tissue and organ with Chi, imagine that the body needs 1200 watts of electricity daily. Everything we eat becomes electricity or Chi, however if our food chains are loaded with chemicals and impurities, we might only consume the equivalent of 300 watts of electricity.

If each meridian automatically divided the 300 watts between them resulting in a 25% of delivery of our optimum need, the meridians would effectively be dimmed down, just like a soft light in your living room. The body would not have the energy required to function normally and maintain itself. In such a situation, one is forever tired, lethargic and often has aches and pains throughout the body. However, the meridian system might decide to divide the 300 watts differently, resulting in some of the meridians having more supply while others struggle due to energy starvation. We find that we are heading for an 'electrical blackout' – a serious disorder or malfunction.

If we take the case of the lung meridian, we could be suffering from arthritis in the thumbs, pain along the arm and even skin conditions along the path of the meridian, as well as pain in front of the shoulder blade. If we do not take notice of these warnings and understand that they are signs of a particular meridian struggling due to vital energy starvation, we may find that we are heading for congestions within our internal meridian, ending with serious and chronic conditions.

While we may go to our doctor and hand over the responsibility for treating the condition by numbing or suppressing it with medication, this may only give a temporary illusion of well-being. Since the internal lung meridian passes through the lungs and part of the colon, if we ignore the warning signs we may end up with a serious asthma attack, difficulty in breathing or ongoing infections within our respiratory system, simply because the Chi has diminished to such a degree that the lungs cannot function properly. (Each meridian and their internal implications is discussed in detail in chapter 4.)

Stress

'The mass of men leads lives of quiet desperation.'

HENRY DAVID THOREAU

Stress is one of the most commonly used words today but stress is not new to the human condition. It has always been present, but is now more prevalent as the pressure and demands of the 21st century take their toll. The word 'stress' is derived from the Latin word stringere that means 'to draw tight'. The modern word 'uptight' accurately describes the response to stress.

The stress reaction is a primitive response to a threatening or danger-ous situation, and has been of essential importance in ensuring the continued survival of the human species. Man is the product of thou-sands of years of evolution. Our survival has depended on quick physical responses to dangers and the stress reaction is commonly referred to as the 'fight-or-flight' reaction. In primitive times, this burst of energy was utilized in physical activity such as a life-or-death strug-gle or a quick dash to safety. Today these responses are largely unacceptable or inappropriate.

Until recently, it was believed that all stress was a result of external forces exerting pressure on an individual. However, this does not explain why, when confronted by similar situations, one person will react calm-ly while another may be completely devastated. More recent theories emphasize that the stress response depends on the interaction between people and their environment. The intensity of the stress experience is determined by how people feel they can cope with an identified threat.

The hormonal and chemical defence mechanisms that evolved over the centuries as a means of protection have been retained, but today they have little outlet. The inability to express a physical response to a stressful situation means that our natural instincts are suppressed and this can cause dire harm.

But what exactly are the physiological effects of stress? When confronted by a situation we perceive as threatening, our thoughts regarding ourselves and the situation trigger two branches of the central nervous system – the sympathetic and parasympathetic systems.

The sympathetic nervous system initiates involuntary responses designed to activate all the major systems of the body. The first response is a flood of hormone secretions. The hypothalamus, when recognizing a danger, triggers the pituitary gland. This gland releases hormones which cause the adrenal glands to intensify the output of adrenaline and nor-adrenaline into the bloodstream. These two hormones mimic the actions of nervous stimulation in a number of organs in the body. Although any number of factors can trigger the adrenocortical stress reaction, the response itself is always the same. It involves the release from the adrenal glands of specific hormones, mainly the corticosteroids, which in turn mobilize the body against invading germs or foreign proteins and enhance one's level of arousal. The stress response always activates the immune system.

The stress chemicals induce physiological changes designed to improve performance. Blood supply to the brain is increased, initially improving judgement and decision-making. The heart speeds up and fuel is released into the bloodstream from glucose, fats or stored blood sugar to provide additional energy. More blood is sent to the muscles to allow for instant action. Breathing rate and function improve as air passages relax. A sense of stimulation is produced and blood pressure rises. Because digestion and excretion are not considered high priorities in a 'dangerous' situation, adrenaline causes vascular constriction, which reduces the flow of blood to the stomach and intestine. Blood vessels dilate in some areas and constrict in others; for example, blood is drained from the skin to make it available for use in other areas such as the muscles.

When the body prepares for 'fight-or-flight', it is ready for a short burst of heightened activity. In modern society, many factors can trigger this response, but few can be dealt with by a short burst of activity. Stress situations are often continuous so stress responses are semi-permanently on red alert, but physical release is usually unacceptable, so the responses are suppressed – a situation which cannot be maintained safely for too long. The stress build-up eventually explodes internally, knocks the body systems out of balance and causes extreme physical and mental exhaustion.

The role of the parasympathetic nervous system is to relax the body after a stressful encounter. However, if a person is subject to continual stress, it becomes more difficult to activate the parasympathetic reaction. If the stress situation continues unabated, the body weakens and becomes more susceptible to a variety of diseases.

Long-term adrenal stimulation with no discharge of energy will deplete essential minerals and vitamins from the system, for example vitamins B and C, which are vital for the functioning of the immune system.[1] This will result in lowered resistance and increased susceptibility to diseases directly related to the immune system such as AIDS (in persons who are HIV-positive) and ME (myalgic encephalomyelitis). Long-term adrenal accumulation can also affect blood pressure and cause a build-up of fatty substances on blood vessel walls, as well as damaging the functioning of the digestive system.

When an organism faces continual or repeated stress, the response system enters the chronic phase during which resistance declines below normal and eventually becomes exhausted. Several diseases result directly from this stage, but the most important effect is a decrease in the body's ability to fight infection and cancer.[2]

Everyone is confronted daily with potentially stressful situations. Our vulnerability to stress can be influenced by life events which cause undue emotional strain. Emotional distress is one resistance-lowering factor. Another important factor, according to some health professionals, is the impact of major life changes. A majority of illnesses are preceded by a constellation of significant events in our lives and future health or disease can be forecast by evaluating these events. The greater the number of life changes, the more serious the oncoming illness.[3]

Enormous changes have been inflicted on and instigated by man in the last four decades in Western society. The rapid technological and social change exerts extreme pressure on humanity. To quote from Alvin Toffler's Future Shock:

> 'There are discoverable limits to the amount of change that the human organism can absorb, by endlessly accelerating these limits, we may submit masses of men to demands they simply cannot tolerate.'[4]

Life changes are a determining factor in stress-related illnesses, but the extent to which the events lead to ill health will depend to a large degree on a person's capacity to cope with stress. The way an individual perceives a situation dramatically affects the stress response experienced. It is not so much the actual ability to cope with a situation that matters as the individual's perception of his ability to cope.

It is believed that up to 80% of modern diseases have stress-related backgrounds. These include hypertension, high blood pressure, coronary thrombosis, heart attack, migraine, hay fever and allergies, asthma, peptic ulcers, constipation, colitis, rheumatoid arthritis, menstrual difficulties, nervous dyspepsia, flatulence and indigestion, hyperthyroidism (overactive thyroid gland), diabetes mellitus, skin disorders, tuberculosis and depression.

We may not be able to alter the stress situations in life, but we can alter how we cope. Natural healing techniques, relaxation techniques, meditation, diet and exercise can all help control or decrease the stress response and thereby lessen one's susceptibility to stress related diseases.

Chi and stress

As we have seen, stress has many angles. However, taking into account that the meridians and all our cellular systems are fuelled with Chi, it is evident that stress can be related to the lack of Chi, or the manner in which the Chi 'performs'. For example, when we eat too many sugar-loaded foodstuffs we put stress on our pancreas that has to work harder than expected. The result might be congestions along the spleen/pancreas meridian, so creating pain in the knees, a painful menstrual cycle with pre-menstrual stress, or swollen sore lateral breasts. At other times, the quality of our food might stress our liver functions and instead of receiving Chi from the metabolized food, the liver might need more Chi in the digesting processes, leading to a Chi deficit. This imbalance may trigger off an outburst of anger or depression that many may label as stress-related – and therefore be blamed on an external rather than an internal factor.

Applying Knowledge of the Five Elements

'The highest wisdom has but one science, the science of the whole, the science explaining the whole of creation and man's place in it.'
LEO TOLSTOY

'A theory is the more impressive the greater is the simplicity of its premises, the more different are the kinds of things it relates, and more extended is its range of applicability.'

ALBERT EINSTEIN

Nowhere in reflexology do these statements hold more relevance than in the connection that exists between the meridians, the Five Elements and the feet. Ancient Chinese philosophy established the five basic elements of fire, earth, metal, water and wood found in the universe, and consequently also in man. The importance was realized of a nourishing and controlling cycle between the elements in order to maintain harmony (see pages 30–31).

Each of these elements relates to a pair of meridians. There are 12 meridians found in the body. Each of them is named according to the organ or system it represents and they are arranged in pairs, which are interdependent. The pairs in their interdependence represent yin and yang (see page 38).

While the Five Elements describe the interrelationship of man and nature, modern man believes he can control the natural processes of change – with a detriment to himself and the planet Earth. As we know, man has distorted our food chains and interfered with the importance of nature. Throughout the Western world, the consequences of man trying to control rather than flow with natural changes continue to have devastating results. Family units are increasingly fragmented; countries go to war to attempt to wrest control; mankind is killing the life force of the sea, and the animal kingdom; and mankind itself is showing strong signs of reduced fertility.

When a person is suffering from the symptoms of malnutrition or toxicity, they will go to a medical doctor where they are told that they suffer from a condition that is causing them their pain and suffering. The condition will have a name such as hypoglycaemia, chronic fatigue syndrome, fibromyalgia, arthritis, sciatica, or whatever the current 'fashionable' disease is at that time. They are then given a prescription for sleeping pills, muscle relaxants or anti-inflammatory medication. Subsequently, they will go through test after test: CAT scans, MRI scans, X-rays, bone scans, urine exams, etc. Neurologists, rheumatologists, orthopaedists, endocrinologists and even chiropractors may examine them. No one will have the same opinion and nothing will be sure to help.[5]

Taking a fresh look at the concept of the Five Elements might help us to understand our life paths and take stronger individual responsibilities for transformation, which not only harmonizes our body systems, but brings about an alteration benefiting our children and their future generations.

A New Look at Five Element Theory

In the past decade, reflexology has carved a respected niche for itself in the realm of holistic healing techniques. People of all ages and from all walks of life have discovered the positive effects to be derived from foot manipulation. The increasing demand for reflexology is proof of its escalating popularity and the pace at which reflexology has been, and is, expanding throughout the Western world is proof of its efficacy. In South Africa, the profession has gained statutory recognition and is now a registered modality within the health professions. The main objective of reflexology is to help people attain and maintain a better state of health and well-being. It does not promise to be a magic panacea for all ills, but there is no longer any doubt that reflexology has an important role to play in the future of health care worldwide.

The remarkable results attained through reflexology stem from the amazing therapeutic potential present in the feet. Some schools of thought recommend stimulating hand reflexes, as well as foot reflexes. Reflexes of body parts are mapped out on the hands in a fashion similar to those on the feet. Massaging the hands may elicit some positive effect, but nothing as powerful as the effect of foot massage. The reason for this is that the six larger meridians – those that actually penetrate major organs, the stomach, spleen/pancreas, liver, gall bladder, kidney and bladder meridians – all begin or end in the toes. The external pathways of the meridians represented in the hands – the heart, small intestine, triple burner, circulation, large intestine and lungs, although associated with specific organs (apart from the triple burner and circulation), do not actually penetrate any major organs.

Hands, like feet, may be afflicted by deformities, but this is due largely to arthritic complaints. Often the same fingers on both hands will be afflicted – for example, the index fingers. All problems on the hands, such as warts, eczema and nail disorders should be assessed as an imbalance along a meridian. As the external pathways of the six hand meridians do not penetrate any major organs – only sensory organs in the facial area – the imbalances, which manifest on the hands, should be weighed up as the result of congestions relating to the major organs and their meridians.

When the concept of the Five Elements is introduced, the scenario becomes even more interesting. The six meridians in the hands are related to two elements – fire and metal. The fire element is represented in the heart, small intestine, circulation and triple burner meridians; and the metal element in the large intestine and lung meridians. The six meridians in the feet represent the wood element in the liver and gall bladder meridians; the water element in the kidney and bladder meridians; and the earth element in the stomach and spleen/pancreas meridians.

When we correlate the elements with body functions and nutrition, the importance of correct nourishment becomes more evident. The earth is central to our physical existence. We derive all physical nourishment from Mother Earth. Internally, the stomach and spleen/pancreas are the equivalent of the Earth. To more fully understand this theory, see figure

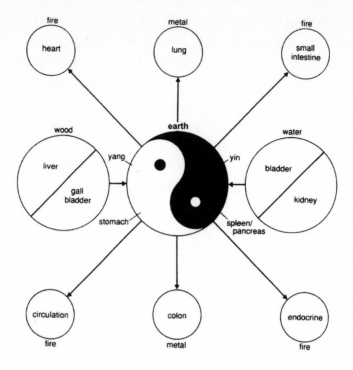

Fig. 1 A new look at the five element theory

1. You will notice that I have placed the earth element in the centre to relate to the yin/yang symbol of perfect balance. The stomach and its meridian control digestion, and the spleen and pancreas and their combined meridian control the distribution of Chi energy released from food when it is digested. If the stomach does not hold and digest food, the spleen/pancreas cannot transform it and transport its essence (see page 90). They are interdependent meridians, and work together more closely than any of the other meridians.

Earth is special among the elements, because it is the source of them, the centre from which they arise – as is the planet Earth to our physical existence. Each of the elements is in constant relationship with the earth element, coming to life and dying within her realm. It has been written that the earth is womb and tomb, the beginning and the end in the never-ending cycle of life, death and rebirth.

Within earth we find water – the rivers, seas, springs; metal in the forms of minerals, gems and fuel (coal); and wood in the plant life. Relating this to meridians – the stomach meridian (earth) penetrates the liver (wood), the kidneys (water) and the lungs and large intestine (metal).

If you refer back to figure 1 you will observe that the wood element is placed on one side of the earth element, and the water element on the other. To balance the earth element (stomach and spleen/pancreas), we must obtain the correct nutrition from the plant kingdom – the wood element. Plants, which have absorbed nutrients from the earth and flourished in sunlight, are saturated with vital Chi energy. This energy is easy to distribute by our meridians into our body organs and cellular systems. In addition to this, we must also have the correct quantity and quality of liquid – the water element –for the digestion and absorption of the food.

The earth element – our stomach and spleen/pancreas – may be related to a compost heap in the garden. If we add plastic, glass or concrete to the compost, these will not metabolize and so be recycled once more as nourishment for the earth. Rather, they add to the pollution of the earth and become non bio-degradable objects. For many, these processes are obvious, but surprisingly few take notice that the food types (wood element), as well as liquids (water element) that we consume daily contain many non bio-degradable chemicals that congest our cells, tissues and organs, as well as our meridians. The additives in many modern foods and liquids combine to form a lethal cocktail. Man and earth are not intended to metabolize inorganic foodstuffs. If we continue at this rate we will soon be positively non-biodegradable. Some additives found in commercially produced food-stuffs include:

- Piperonal – used in place of vanilla – is a chemical used to treat lice.
- Diethyl glucol – a cheap chemical used as an emulsifier instead of eggs – is used in antifreeze and paint removers.

- Butyraldehyde – used in nut-flavoured foods – is one of the ingredients in rubber cement.
- Amyl acetate – used for banana flavour – is also an oil-paint solvent.
- Ethyl acetate – used for pineapple flavour – is also used as a cleaner for leather and textiles.
- Aldehyde C17 – flavours cherry ice-cream – is an inflammable liquid used in aniline dyes, plastic and rubber.

In chapter 4 you will learn that amongst others the stomach and spleen/pancreas preside over the fatty connective tissues of the body. It is probable that the non-biodegradable chemicals, which the body does not metabolise nor eliminate, are stored in these fatty connective tissues. It is no coincidence that modern society is having an epidemic with both weight problems and diabetes and does not seem to find the correct life-style or understanding in dealing with these global issues.

Apart from adding foods to our stomach (earth element) we also add liquids (water element); however, it is known that too much added water to compost heaps creates an unpleasant rotting effect that invites parasites, rather than a good ecosystem of earthworms. We do not always appreciate that we add plenty of liquids to our digestive system in the form of natural foods. These natural fluids contain many of the minerals that keep the sodium and potassium salt balance of the tissue fluid in our cellular system intact. (See the section on the cell on pages 64–68.) Nonetheless, if we eat mainly processed foods our cells will dehydrate and the cellular system will become imbalanced, the effect being felt in the form of congestions and signs of thirst.

During the first phase of the digestive process – oxygen and carbon dioxide are released (gases: metal element). These processes happen in all cells, but the lungs and large intestine (metal element) are the organs where the main exchanges occur, hence in figure 1 the lungs (metal element) are shown above and the large intestine (metal element) below

the stomach, as an image of the body. The second phase in the digestive process is the creation of energy, which in the compost heap can
be related to heat (fire element) and in the body to our Chi or zest for
life (fire element).

It is interesting to note that the six meridians that are found in the
hands and relate to the metal and fire elements, represent the organs
that seem to correspond to many of the diseases of the modern society of today. By taking a closer look at the six organs or systems and
relating them to modern disorders and imbalances we might witness
the correlation of 'input versus output' in regards to our food intake.
We see that many people now suffer from disorders of the respiratory
system, such as asthma, bronchitis, sinusitis and ongoing nasal congestions which represent the metal element and therefore the exchange of
oxygen and carbon dioxide. Many nutritional experts today consider
that we are not getting enough oxygen through our food, and yet we
continue to drink carbon-loaded fizzy drinks. Furthermore, the most
misused remedy, that of laxatives, shows evidence that the partner –
the large intestines – have major problems. The large intestines symbol-
ize the main compost heap, and a friendly bacterium to help keeping
the ecology balanced is a must, just like the earthworms in the compost. However, many people suffer from a bloated, yeast-congested
ecology, showing evidence of unfriendly parasites that eat away the
minimal nourishment that is left, leaving behind an unhealthy non-
metabolized 'compost'.

On figure 1, the four meridians linked to the fire element have been
placed in four corners of the figure. Each of these fire meridians has an
internal branch meridian going to the heart. (See also the section on
external versus internal meridians, page 48.) I am trying to convey here
a strong message – that of looking after our fire within, since it is this
fire that keeps us alive and gives us the zest for life. If our internal
'compost heap' has no nutritional value, how can we fuel and keep our
fire alive?

More than 25% of the population of the modern society will suffer from heart-related problems. The partner organ is the small intestine and its meridian, which gives evidence that the function of our heart is directly linked to the nutritional absorption from our small intestine. This raises the possibility that we may suffer from malnutrition from lack of Chi – even though we eat plenty of foods.

The circulation and the triple burner meridians, symbolizing the function of our blood and the endocrine system, are the two other systems relating to the fire element. Many blood and circulatory disorders are now on the increase in modern society – such as, hardening of the arteries, cholesterol, leukaemia, varicose veins, as well as inflammation. With regard to the endocrine system, it would be difficult to find a person who is not somehow affected by a hormonal imbalance. One symptom of this is evidence of a strong increase of infertility in both males and females.

Feeding Your Stomach/Compost to make Fire/Chi

There is a distinct possibility that we are destroying our own earth (stomach and spleen/pancreas). Few can honestly say they enjoy vibrant, boundless health, free from niggling aches, pains, allergies and mood swings. In place of the dynamic energy, which is our birthright, we have been conditioned to accept health as simply the absence of disease. Western nations spend millions on caring for the sick, and thousands of man-hours are lost every year through minor illness and impaired performance. Much of this needless suffering and expense could be alleviated if just a fraction of the money spent on remedial health care was channelled into education on diet, nutrition and prevention. The one area of our lives over which most of us have total control is our diet and lifestyle. It is probably the most important factor in the maintenance of health – and the greatest cause of the development of disease. The human body is created and maintained from the food we eat. Because we are made of energy fields, we are dependent on the energies we absorb from food. We should therefore eat foods compatible with our energy needs that will stimulate rather than obstruct the free flow of Chi in the body. The value of plant energy is mentioned by world-renowned healer and psychic Edgar Cayce in the book The Hidden Laws of the Earth:

> 'Energy values in the food we eat are of great importance. Where does the energy in our food come from? The solar energy reaching the earth is absorbed by the leaves of plants. In the plants it joins with water, minerals and nitrogen compounds which the roots have sucked up from the ground and also carbonic acid, a gas which man breathes out as a waste product and which has been gathered by the plant from the air. The sun's energy is transferred into a new energy, and the plant energy becomes fixed in a state of rest and is then potential energy. In other words, chemical vital energy is produced by plants from solar energy. Man eats the plants and then utilizes the chemical vital energy. Food from plants is higher in potential energy than that from animal products. Eating animal products is eating the energy second-hand.'

Nutrition is involved in every bodily activity and diet furnishes the raw materials or nutrients required for the synthesis of chemical substances indispensable to the body's growth, maintenance and repair. Unfortunately, the modern trend is towards food empty of essential nutrients and we have become divorced from our natural instincts. Animals instinctively know which plants and grasses are good for them and which are bad, and will choose to eat those beneficial to their health and avoid those which are detrimental. However, we humans are rather perverse and have developed a tendency to eat food that is bad for us based purely on sensuous taste and pleasure value. This tendency can be cited as one of the major causes of disease today.

The Five Elements and the Cell

The basic unit of life is the cell. Cells all require the same nutrients, such as glucose (or blood sugar), amino acids, vitamins, minerals and enzymes. All cells use oxygen to burn fuel and give off carbon dioxide and metabolic wastes, which are delivered to the fluids surrounding them as end products of chemical reactions. Cells live in a watery environment known as interstitial fluid or tissue fluid. This fluid consists of quantities of potassium and sodium salts – outside is a high concentration of potassium and little sodium; inside the balance is reversed. Biochemists are steadily expanding their comprehension of the phenomenon of the transfer of electricity across cell membranes. These electric impulses are carried along the nerves as a result of changes in the quantities of potassium and sodium. From this viewpoint, the cell can be looked upon as a small electric battery and all functions of the human body are electro-chemical in their operations. In this way, each cell benefits from a correct chemical balance in your body, or homeostasis, and each cell contributes its share toward the maintenance of homeostasis.

The chemistry of body fluids must be balanced in order for the process of fermentation to function normally. This requires a pH acid/alkaline balance. Normal blood pH has a very small window of normal range – it must range between 7.35 and 7.45. This means that there will be an adequate quantity of oxygen in the blood. Even a slight decrease in blood pH will result in lower oxygen levels and, therefore, in the cells. And this slight drop in pH will mark the beginning of a disease state. For water or fluids to be most effective in our body, it is necessary that they contain the ionized minerals required to nourish and protect cells, including bacteria. They should have a slightly higher pH, which is necessary to assure that the body fluids do not become and remain over acidic, resulting in deterioration. However, the contamination of our environment (such as toxic wastes and chemical additives to food and drinking water) has depleted the required minerals from our foods, resulting in metabolic disturbances, and creating a more rapid disease and ageing process to occur.

Together, cells make up tissues, and tissues make up organs. Organs make up systems that again make up an organism such as a human being. In order for the organism to remain alive and healthy, these systems, organs, tissues and cells must obtain 90 basic nutrients necessary for normal function daily. These essential elements are obtained from our environment in the form of what we eat and what we breathe.

The Five Elements as a Cell

On the next page you will find two illustrations – one the same as figure 2 on page 30 (Generating/control cycle); however around the figures a circle has been added taking the profile of a membrane around the cell. The interaction within the Five Elements can be perceived in the same manner as the interaction within a cell and therefore the generating and controlling cycles. All things contain all Five Elemental energies in various proportions. In the second illustration, I have replaced the names of the Five Elements to attempt to Westernize the concept, so making it easier to understand and therefore apply.

The ultimate task of each cell is to convert nutrients into energy – or Chi. The ultimate task of the Five Elements is to create a well-balanced fire that will continue maintaining life at its optimum.

In place of wood (gall bladder/liver), which clearly represents the plant world which ultimately feeds all living creatures including man – hence being associated with active functions and growth – we should read 'food chains'. In place of earth, representing the stomach and spleen/pancreas meridians and their organs, as well as a neutral state of balance, we should read acid/alkaline (base) balance, and also blood sugar balance. Nutrition is the key to stabilizing the levels of blood

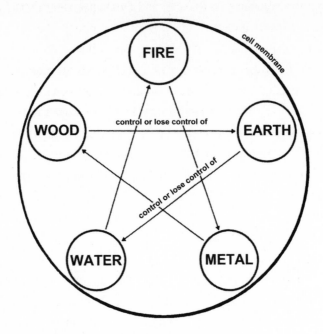

Fig. 2a The Five Elements as a cell (1)

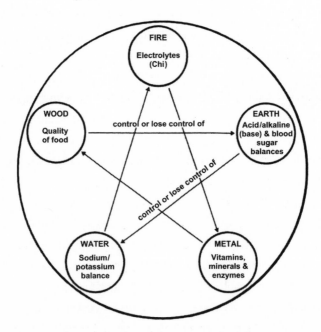

Fig. 2b The Five Elements as a cell (2)

sugar and acid/alkaline balance. After a meal, glucose from the breakdown of food (wood element) is absorbed through the wall of the intestine into the bloodstream giving rise to a high level of glucose in the blood. The body uses what it immediately needs for energy and then produces insulin from the pancreas to lower the level of excess glucose. Glucose that is not used immediately is transformed into glycogen and stored in the liver and muscles to be used later. The glucose level in the blood then reduces to normal.

With regard to metal (lung/large intestine), relating to a declining state within the elements, this action should translate to vitamins, minerals and enzymes. An enzyme is defined as a biological catalyst; it enters into a chemical reaction but does not become a part of the action itself. The enzyme is considered the 'brain' of the cell. Each cell in our body has its own enzyme, and all reactions that occur in each cell are dictated and controlled by the enzyme. Enzyme failure is the ultimate cause of disease. As an alternative to water (bladder/kidney), we need to substitute the vital sodium/potassium salt balance within the cellular system. The sodium/potassium salt balance is what keeps the fluid in a balanced proportion inside and outside the cell walls. The water element reflects those functions that have reached a state of maximum rest, and are preparing to change direction into activity. Fire (heart/small intestine and circulation/endocrine or triple burner) is more obscure and can have many translations explaining the same outcome – being Chi, zest for life, life-force or, in medical terms, our balance of electrolytes. The fire element includes functions that have reached a maximum state of activity and that are about to decline to a resting period.

In our new interpretation, the interactions (control or loss of control) between the elements will read as follows:

• The quality and quantity of food (wood element), control or lose control of the acid/alkaline and the blood sugar balances (earth element).

- The acid/alkaline and blood sugar balances (earth element) control or lose control of the sodium/potassium balance within the cellular system (water element), which again control or lose control of the electrolytes in the body (fire element).
- A primary purpose of kidneys (water element) is to balance electrolytes in blood (fire element).
- Electrolytes are the key to unlock energy flow in a cell. They strike the sparks of electric fire that make life happen. Minerals are needed to keep this 'battery' in a cell going, and to enable the cell to hold a charge. Without minerals – without the right electrolytes in correct ratios – cells weaken, become vulnerable to parasites and even die. The link between electrolytes (fire element) and minerals, vitamins and enzymes (metal element) can consequently be better understood.
- The same goes with the reality that the quality and quantity of minerals, vitamins and enzymes (metal element) have a profound influence on the quality of our food chains (wood element) – back to the beginning!

This description of the Five Elements and their meridians has been included to provide some 'food for thought' and help explain the theories contained in this book. It emphasizes the relevance of the theory that the potent positive effects derived from reflexology are linked to the presence of meridians in the feet – meridians that relate to the three central elements of earth, wood and water, and which all penetrate the major body organs, whose functions are specifically associated with nutrition, digestion and distribution. The six meridians in the hands reflect the results of the interaction between wood, earth and water, giving evidence of potential imbalances. Applying therapeutic pressure to the feet stimulates not only the reflexes and related body parts, but also the six larger meridians, thereby helping to clear congestions along all the meridians and activate the circulation of vital Chi energy, which revitalizes the whole body.

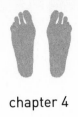

chapter 4

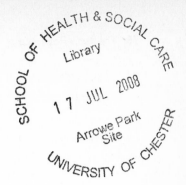
the 5 elements and their 12 meridians

'There are no miracles, only unknown laws.'

SAINT AUGUSTINE

In ancient China, people understood the importance of nature and many healing arts were based on knowledge and insight gleaned from it. They realized that as nature around them went through processes of change, the same patterns also occurred within man.

The Chinese established five basic elements – wood, fire, earth, metal and water – that interact in a creative cycle to form all other substances. The Five Elements do not refer to material elements, but rather to conditions or states.

Each element is associated with inner organs and these are divided into two classes. The first are the six organs whose function is nutrition and excretion:

- stomach,
- large intestine,
- bladder,
- gall bladder,

- small intestine,
- triple burner.

The other six organs are associated with energy circulation, storage and distribution:

- spleen/pancreas,
- lungs,
- kidneys,
- liver,
- heart,
- circulation/pericardium.

The triple burner and circulation/pericardium are not organs in the sense of Western physiology, but fall into this category in Chinese medicine.

The correspondences

Apart from the organs, each element is identified with other specific correspondences. These include season, climate, taste, colour, emotion and sound. Extreme reactions to any of these may indicate an imbalance in the related element. All these correspondences indicate only the predominant element – nothing is wholly any one element to the exclusion of others. Every thing in existence contains all five elements but one element so predominates that it is named accordingly.[1] Careful study of these will clarify their aid as diagnostic tools. In this section we will look at symbolic parallels, and some of the more obvious, easy-to-read correspondences that can aid in diagnosis.

The Chinese believed that climate had a profound effect on Chi. Weather affects our lives, sometimes beneficially, but often disruptively. While we are able to adapt to our environment to a certain extent, a sudden change in climate can cause an imbalance within our meridians. External

FIVE ELEMENTS CATEGORIZATION CHART

ELEMENT	METAL	EARTH	FIRE	WATER	WOOD
SEASON	Autumn	Late Summer	Summer	Winter	Spring
EMOTION	Grief, Worry	Sympathy, Compassion, Desire	Joy, Happiness	Fears, Phobias, Anxiety	Anger
TIME	Lung 3 am – 5 am Large Intestine 5 am – 7 am	Stomach 7 am – 9 am Spleen/Pancreas 9 am – 11 am	Heart 11 am – 1 pm Small Intestine 1 pm – 3 pm Pericardium 7 pm – 9 pm Triple Burner 9 pm – 11 pm	Bladder 3 pm – 5 pm Kidney 5 pm – 7 pm	Gall bladder 11 pm – 1 am Liver 1 am – 3 am
SOUND	Crying, Weeping	Singing	Laughing	Groaning	Shouting
TISSUES	Skin, Body Hair	Fatty Connective Tissue	Blood Vessels	Bone, Teeth, Bone Marrow	Muscles, Ligaments, Tendons
EXTN. PHYS. MANIF.	Skin, Body Hair	Flesh	Complexion	Quality of Head Hair	Nails
SENSE ORGANS	Nose	Mouth/Lips	Tongue	Ears	Eyes
BODY FLUID	Mucous	Saliva	Perspiration	Spittle around Teeth	Tears
FLAVOUR	Pungent, Spicy	Sweet	Bitter	Salty	Sour
SMELL	Rotten	Sickening, Cloying	Scorched	Putrid	Rancid
CLIMATE	Dry	Humidity	Heat	Cold	Wind
COLOURS	White	Yellow	Red	Blue	Green

forces experienced in excess can cause illness, and this is why it is important to take particular care of health at times of season change. An adverse reaction to, or preference for, a specific climate or season is important in traditional diagnosis.[2]

Emotion is also important. When in a healthy state, human beings should be able to feel and express all of the five emotions as appropriate. Every illness or imbalance is bound up with an emotion. The sound of our voice reflects our emotion. This can be perceived as a subtle tone in a person's voice or a vociferous expression of emotion, such as shouting in anger or crying. Excessive or deficient emotion or sound can indicate a specific energy imbalance.

With regard to taste, each flavour has an effect on energy. The combination of the five tastes ensures balance. An excess of one flavour can have an injurious effect, yet each element can be strengthened if the right flavour is prescribed for it.[3] The Nei Ching states:

> 'If people pay attention to the five flavours and blend them well, their bones will remain straight, their muscles will remain tender and young, breath and blood will circulate freely, the pores will be in fine texture, and consequently breath and bones will be filled with the essence of life.'[4]

Any aversion to or obsession with a specific taste will indicate an imbalance in the related element.

In a similar way, a specific colour preference or dislike can provide useful information regarding element balance. Colour can also be perceived in the face. If Chi is flowing harmoniously within each element and among the elements, the face will not show any predominant colour. If one of the elements is imbalanced, the colour associated with it will show on the face. This is not skin colour, but rather a subtle hue coming from the face.

Other element correspondences relating specifically to body functions – sense organs, fluid secretions, tissue weakness and external physical manifestation – are closely related to organ function. Any disturbances related to these correspondences clearly indicate specific energy imbalances within a particular element.

Muscles and their Relationship to the Meridians

Muscular symptoms are important and revealing in relating problems to causes. Muscular problems are often the main reason a patient seeks assistance and treatment. The muscles also relate to specific meridians and organs, and understanding this relationship can enable you to assist the deficient organ back to an optimum state of health, thereby eliminating muscle problems.

The muscles form the flesh of the body. There are two types of muscle: voluntary muscle, made up of striped or cross-banded tissue, and involuntary muscle comprising smooth cells without cross stripes. Each voluntary muscle consists of a large number of separate fibres. These are bound together in bundles by a sheath of connective tissue called the perimysium. The whole muscle is then covered by a sheet of fibrous tissue called fascia, and is connected to the bone by tendons.

When stimulated, each muscle fibre contracts – gets shorter and thicker. As the muscle passes over one or more joints, this contraction pulls one bone towards the other, thus producing movement at the joint. The type of movement depends on the position and shape of the muscles and the type of joint they cross.

A muscle must have an adequate blood and nerve supply before it can contract. It receives glucose and oxygen from the blood. The nerve supplies the impulse, which initiates a series of chemical changes involving glucose and oxygen. These changes release the energy which make the

muscles contract.[5] When movement is required, carbohydrates are broken down, oxygen is carried to muscles in the bloodstream and a series
of chemical changes occur, which release energy and produce heat. The
energy makes the muscle contract and the heat helps to maintain the
body temperature at 37°C. The waste produced by muscle action is carbon dioxide and water, and these are conveyed mostly by the blood to
the lungs and breathed out, although the skin, the bladder and the
bowel also excrete some of the water. The muscles become inactive if
the blood and nerve supply is interrupted.

The assumption used to be that the main causes of backache and associated disorders were muscles which were either in spasm or too taut,
thus affecting the spine. However, Dr George Goodheart, the founder of
the practice known as 'Applied Kinesiology', began to work on a different idea: that it might not be the muscle spasm or tautness that was
the problem, but rather that it was 'weak muscles' on the opposite side
of the body which caused the normal muscles to appear tight. Combining Eastern ideas about energy flow with his own chiropractic
techniques, he discovered that the tests used in kinesiology to determine the relative muscle strength and tone over the range of
movement of the joints could also reveal the balance of energy in each
of the body's systems. Further research led him to identify the relationship between each specific muscle group, the particular organs and the
meridians of acupuncture.

Although in reflexology we do not practise muscle testing to ascertain
weakness in the body, this knowledge can be useful to reflexologists. For
example, a person with headaches on the bladder meridian may also
suffer calf cramps. The calf muscles (soleus and gastrocnemius) are both
related to the bladder and its meridian, confirming an imbalance.
Another form of headache may be associated with the gall bladder
meridian. The person may have related symptoms such as nausea, hip
pain or frozen shoulder. The shoulder muscle (anterior deltoid) is related to the gall bladder and its meridian. I have also seen patients with

weight problems who are unable to shed the weight from their thigh or calf muscles. The calf muscles (gastrocnemius and soleus) and thigh muscles (sartorius and gracilis) are related to the triple burner (endocrine) meridian, thus indicating a hormonal imbalance as the cause of the weight problem. Muscle-related disorders associated with the kidney meridian are problems with the neck/shoulder area and the hip/pelvic area. Many people complain of neck tension and believe the cause merely to be tension. However, it could be the result of overloading the kidneys and bladder. If the kidneys do not efficiently eliminate toxins, they may be stored in the neck or hip regions. If this is not corrected the toxins remain in these muscles and eventually begin to eat away at the bone structure.

From this it is clear that muscle problems can indicate organ imbalance. This is further evidenced by an interesting case history. A male in his early sixties had suffered a frozen shoulder for six months. His doctor offered little hope of improvement and the only relief he could give was cortisone injections. When he came for reflexology treatment, I enquired about the state of his gall bladder, and was told that it had been removed during the war. The doctors had been puzzled at the time, as the organ appeared quite healthy, apart from being slightly enlarged. The patient then mentioned a 'souvenir' from the war – a bullet behind his knee – in the popliteus muscle, which relates to the gall bladder. In fact, this may have been the cause of the frozen shoulder and the enlarged gall bladder. The muscles related to the meridians are illustrated in the detailed section on meridians.

THE METAL ELEMENT

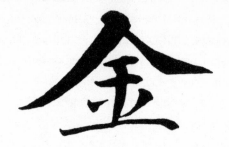

Fig. 1 Metal element

Metal represents the minerals, vitamins and enzymes from the plant world and therefore the quality of our food chains. The metal element can be associated with substance, strength and structure. It provides the main ingredients in systems of communication and provides the substance with which to build communications; it also conducts electricity.[6] Within the cellular system, the function of minerals, vitamins and enzymes is the creation and maintenance of structure and communication which enables our Chi to flow freely. Our lungs communicate between the inner and outer atmospheres and constitute a key organ for our existence. Performing the essential function of respiration, the lungs exchange oxygen and carbon dioxide through the capillaries.

In the human body, the ability to take in food and air, to assimilate and utilize fuel, and then to eliminate waste products are life sustaining aspects of the metal element. Problems with the structure and strength of the body and mind are symptoms of metal imbalance.[7]

The lungs and the large intestine are two areas of our body that must stay clean for their best function, and their functions are often impaired when they are contaminated by the environmental pollutants of cities, by smoking habits and by dietary excess. As we saw earlier (see page 59) modern food chains are frequently corrupted by additives and preservatives and lack most of the essential minerals and enzymes, resulting in the body and mind becoming constipated. Laxatives are now one of the most abused remedies, and communication failure between fellow man has become the biggest dilemma within family units, relationships, work environment, as well as amongst our politicians.

The Lung Meridian

A yin meridian has a descending flow of energy, which runs from the chest to the hand. The lung meridian starts at the clavicle and ends on the back of the thumb towards the index finger (see figure 2).

The Nei Ching states:

> 'The lungs are the symbol of the interpretation and conduct of the official jurisdiction and regulation ... The lungs are the origin of the breath and the dwelling of the animal spirits or inferior soul.'

The lungs and large intestine are partner meridians and both govern elimination. Due to their close relationship, they can directly affect each other; for example, chest problems can be accompanied by large intestine disorders, and vice versa.

Chi from the air outside is inhaled into the lungs where it comes into contact with the Chi inside the body. Healthy lungs and regular even respiration ensures that Chi enters and leaves the body smoothly. An imbalance in the function of this organ and its associated meridian will result in chest problems. Respiratory functions affect all the rhythms of the body, including blood flow. The lungs are also concerned with the movement and transformation of water in the body. They liquefy water vapour and move it down to the kidneys. The secretion of sweat is regulated by the lungs, as they work to scatter water vapour throughout the body to be eliminated via the skin and pores. As the nose and throat

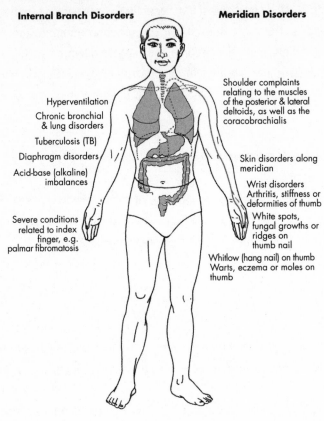

Internal Branch Disorders

Meridian Disorders

Hyperventilation

Chronic bronchial
& lung disorders

Tuberculosis (TB)

Diaphragm disorders

Acid-base (alkaline)
imbalances

Severe conditions
related to index
finger, e.g.
palmar fibromatosis

Shoulder complaints
relating to the muscles
of the posterior & lateral
deltoids, as well as the
coracobrachialis

Skin disorders along
meridian

Wrist disorders
Arthritis, stiffness or
deformities of thumb

White spots,
fungal growths or
ridges on
thumb nail

Whitlow (hang nail) on thumb
Warts, eczema or moles on
thumb

Fig. 2 Lung meridian

are included in the respiratory functions, they too are related to the lungs. The lungs are referred to as the 'delicate organ' as they are most easily influenced by external environmental factors.[8]

Lung meridian congestions

Pain along the course of the meridian; shoulder complaints relating to the muscles of the posterior and lateral deltoids, as well as the coraco-brachialis. Skin disorders along the meridian; wrist disorders, arthritis, stiffness or deformities of the thumb. Any problems occurring on the thumbs and thumbnails, such as white spots, fungal or ridges, whitlow (hang nail), eczema, moles and warts.

Internal branch congestions

Hyperventilation, chronic bronchial and lung disorders, tuberculosis (TB) and diaphragm disorders, as well as hydrochloric acid imbalance. Severe conditions related to index finger, such as palmar fibromatosis.

Muscles associated with the lung meridian

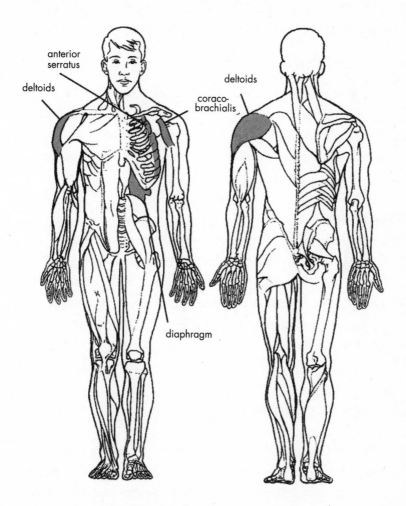

Fig. 3 Muscles associated with the lungs

ANTERIOR SERRATUS

This muscle draws the shoulder blade forward and raises the ribs. Weakness will make it difficult to push things forward with the arms straight, causing the shoulder blades to wing out in the back. It can also affect chest conditions and the diaphragm's ability to regulate breathing.[9]

CORACOBRACHIALIS

This works with the anterior deltoid in straightening the arm when it is held over the head and in flexing the shoulder with the elbow bent, as when combing the hair. They are not usually found to be weak.[10]

DELTOIDS

This is the triangular muscle of the shoulder arising from the clavicle and scapula, with insertion into the humerus. It draws the arm away from the body, lifting the elbow. Weakness will make it difficult to raise the arm. Lung problems such as bronchitis, pleurisy, pneumonia, congestion and flu will usually affect the deltoid.[11]

DIAPHRAGM

The diaphragm is a muscular dome-shaped partition separating the chest cavity from the abdominal cavity. It is the primary muscle used in breathing. A disturbance in the muscle balance of the diaphragm can cause breathing difficulties, hiccups and reduce breath-holding time. There may be digestive disturbances, especially discomfort immediately after eating.[12]

The large intestine/colon meridian

A yang meridian with an ascending flow of energy running from the hand to the head. It receives energy from the lung meridian and transmits it to the stomach meridian. The large intestine meridian starts on the back of the index finger, ascends up the arm and ends next to the nose (see figure 4).

'The large intestine is like the officials who propagate the right way of living and generate evolution and change,' states the Nei Ching. As the 'generator of evolution and change', the correct functioning of this organ is vital to the well-being of the whole body. The large intestine forms the lower part of the digestive tract and is in charge of transporting, transforming and eliminating surplus matter. The important function of elimination of waste material is imperative to the maintenance of health. If this is not carried out effectively, the rest of the system has to cope with an additional load of toxins, which will have a harmful effect on the entire system and cause disharmony throughout the body.

The primary function of the large intestine is the absorption of water, but it also completes the absorption of nutrients and minerals, and houses beneficial bacteria, which help break down food and synthesize vitamins. This organ also forms, stores and eliminates the faeces.

Large intestine meridian congestions

Any problems occurring on the index fingers and nails, such as white spots, fungal or ridges, whitlow (hang nail), eczema, moles and warts. Arthritis, stiffness or deformities of the index fingers, as well as wrist disorders. Stiff and painful forearm, tennis/golfer's elbow, as well as skin disorders along the path of the meridian. Herpes simplex on the lips; disorders of the sense of smelling, as well as bleeding nose (epistaxis), itching or sores in the nose.

Internal branch congestions

Chronic bronchial and lung disorders, weakness of quadratus lumborum muscles and disorders of the ascending and descending colon. 'Referral' pains down the legs.

Internal Branch Disorders   **Meridian Disorders**

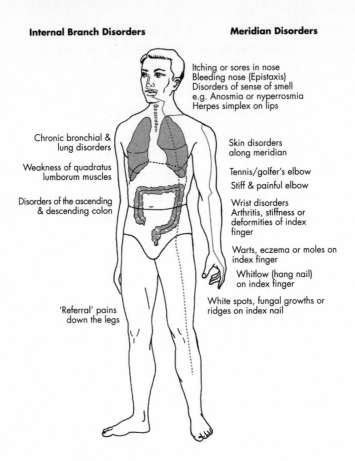

Itching or sores in nose
Bleeding nose (Epistaxis)
Disorders of sense of smell
e.g. Anosmia or nyperrosmia
Herpes simplex on lips

Chronic bronchial &
lung disorders

Weakness of quadratus
lumborum muscles

Disorders of the ascending
& descending colon

Skin disorders
along meridian

Tennis/golfer's elbow

Stiff & painful elbow

Wrist disorders
Arthritis, stiffness or
deformities of index
finger

Warts, eczema or moles on
index finger

Whitlow (hang nail)
on index finger

White spots, fungal growths or
ridges on index nail

'Referral' pains
down the legs

Fig. 4 Large intestine meridian

Muscles related to the large intestine meridian

TENSOR FASCIAE LATAE

This muscle helps flex or bend the thigh, draw it away from the body sideways, and keep it turned in. With weakness, the leg may tend to bow, the thigh turning outward.[13]

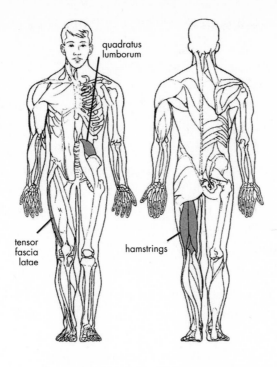

quadratus
lumborum

tensor
fascia
latae

hamstrings

Fig 5. Muscles associated with the large intestine

HAMSTRINGS

These are situated in the back of the thigh. They flex the leg and turn it sideways when the knee is bent. Weakness will cause either a bow-legged or knock-kneed posture. Hamstrings are important in walking.[14]

QUADRATUS LUMBORUM

This flexes the vertebral column sideways, drawing it towards the hip. It assists in the action of the diaphragm in breathing and is a major stabilizing muscle of the lower back. Weakness on one side of the muscle will show in the posture as an elevation of the last rib on the weak side and a curve in the lumbar vertebrae.[15]

The behavioural patterns of the individual with metal element imbalances

THE SEASON: AUTUMN

The metal element relates to autumn – a time of slowing down, harvesting and preparing for winter. It is a time when all things begin to conserve and store nourishment while externally life seems to be fading. As this is true in nature, it is also true in us. If a person cannot harvest and store within themselves the nourishing things that will carry them through the period of austerity, the body and mind will suffer. Maturity or harvesting the life experience is also associated with metal. Generally, we should be harvesting all the natural Chi that we have been eating throughout the summer period, in the form of vegetables, herbs and fruits directly from the garden; however, summer is the time when we may eat more fast foods, pizzas, soda drinks and ice-creams, finding little time or interest in gardening, or preparing and eating fresh organic foods. If this is the case, this may lead to a low immune system, giving rise in early autumn to the first bout of flu or bronchial attack, and ongoing medication continuing into winter and spring. People who detest autumn may be having difficulties in harvesting their own energy. This may show as bowel problems such as diarrhoea, which is an inability to collect the waste for disposal.

THE EMOTION: GRIEF AND WORRY

Emotionally, if energy is circulating as it should, we feel positive and happy. If not, the opposite symptoms – sadness, grief and a tendency to weep – will occur. A person who has gone or is going through a period of grief will often experience bowel problems and/or breathing difficulties, and if the stagnated energy is not shifted by balancing the metal element this can sometimes last a lifetime.

THE TIME OF DAY OF PEAK: LUNGS 3–5 AM; LARGE INTESTINE 5–7 AM

The early hours of the morning are often seen as the 'natural' time of birth – taking in the first breath – as well as the natural time of death – taking one's last breath. However, during the same time, problems within the element might be expressed in the form of an asthma attack or heavy breathing problems. A worrier might start feeling awake and begin stressing about concerns that have yet to happen. First activity in the morning should be the natural time for emptying the bowel – letting go of waste in order to take in new nourishment – if not, the person may become constipated in body and mind.

THE SOUND: WEEPING

This is not necessarily accompanied with real tears, but rather is a sound of tears. For these people even joyful events are tinged with the sound of weeping. Also, a lack of weeping and the inability to cry when appropriate shows evidence of a metal imbalance.

THE TISSUES: SKIN, BODY HAIR

The skin is a third lung and breathes just as surely as the lungs themselves. The skin reflects the condition of the metal element and therefore all skin disorders (such as eczema, dry skin, psoriasis, moles and blemishes) have to be treated as an imbalance within the metal element and consequently a lack of essential vitamins, minerals and enzymes giving strength to these tissues. Even hard calluses on the feet, dry heels and corns should be understood and treated with the primary cause of imbalance in the metal element. In the West, it is not unusual to find asthma accompanied, preceded or followed by some form of eczema.

THE EXTERNAL PHYSICAL MANIFESTATIONS: BODY HAIR, SKIN

Excessive body hair, the loss of body hair (alopecia) and the lack of body hair are evidence of the balance or imbalance of the metal element. The overall skin condition shows the metal element state (for more on this, see 'The Tissues' above).

THE SENSE ORGAN: NOSE

The pathway of the large intestine (colon) meridian ends at the nose, hence the possibility of itching or sores in the nose, bleeding nose (epistaxis) and disorders with the sense of smell – either a loss of the sensation of smell or being over-sensitive to smells. Children with allergies often experience irritations within the nasal cavities and will be seen to move their hands to and fro over the nose.

THE FLUID SECRETION: MUCOUS

Lack of mucous causing dryness of the throat and nose, coughing and difficulty in breathing, or too much mucous causing constant nasal drip and sinus blockage are confirmation of metal imbalances.

THE FLAVOUR/TASTE: SPICY AND PUNGENT

Anyone who eats hot spices knows that the flavour soon 'opens up' the senses, clears the sinuses and makes mucous flow. Also, cheeses, curry, sauces and peppery sorts of foods have a tendency of making too much mucous; both a craving or dislike may confirm an imbalance.

THE SMELL: ROTTEN

When various body organs and their functions have become congested, evidence of the serious condition is often accompanied by a change in body odour that is difficult to describe. Anyone who has worked with very sick people or has been a visitor in a hospital or old age home will recognize each ward as having its own odour. In regards to the metal element, diseases such as tuberculosis, which often present with thick green mucous, have a definite odour of rot, confirming a metal imbalance.

THE CLIMATE: DRY

Often the external weather pattern is blamed for our bodily mishaps and a dry climate can necessitate asthma sufferers to use damp inhalers or move to more damp areas. No weather patterns should make anyone sick – rather we have to adapt with the correct clothing and nutritional intake. A person who complains that dryness is the cause for their illness confirms a metal imbalance.

THE COLOUR: WHITE

A white transparent hue to the face is evidence of an imbalance of Chi energy in the metal element. Children in the developed world suffering from allergies, chest and bowel disorders often demonstrate translucent white faces showing the facial veins. An affinity to the white colour in the use of interior decorating and clothing verifies an imbalance.

THE EARTH ELEMENT

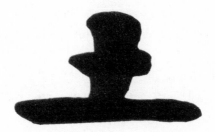

Fig. 6 Earth element

The fertile and stable Earth we know as our 'mother' not only gives us the food we eat – the earth is our support on which we stand and lay ourselves to rest: our womb and our tomb. Being earthy or grounded is having our roots in a solid base. The earth, revolving around its axis to make a day, relates to the cycles in nature, in both man and woman, and is central to all other elements. Earth is special among all the elements, because she is their source. The earth holds the water (streams, rivers and seas) and wood (plant life), the mountains, rocks, minerals being the metal and the essence of it all – the transformation to Chi (fire).

The stomach meridian (earth) penetrates the liver and gall bladder (wood) and the colon and lung (metal), as well as the kidneys (water).

As our life and health revolves around nourishment and the need thereof – an imbalanced rhythm and harmony of the earth element make for all other elements to be affected. Earth deals with the functions of the stomach and the spleen/pancreas and therefore the important acid/alkaline and blood sugar balances. When we lose control of our acid/alkaline balance we lose control of our blood sugar, and vice versa.

The earth element not only refers to the ground on which we stand, but also to a sense of being grounded and rooted within ourselves. People with a strong earth element will be centred, well integrated and feel at home with themselves as well as the outside world, at ease in all situations. People suffering from a deficiency in this element may tend to become obsessed, constantly looking elsewhere for answers and support, and never realize that this must come from their own centre.

The waning and waxing of the moon and its seasons influence the yin and yang energies within the earth element. Those experiencing difficulty with sterility are confirming to the world that their earth is not fertile enough. Problems with conception and birth occur when the earth element has not been prepared and nourished properly. As in nature, if a seed is planted in barren soil that has not been cultivated it will not take root and grow, or if it does it may not come to fruition. The human seeds must be rich and well-balanced if the DNA structures are to bear the journey of life in a healthy, balanced being. The concept of a healthy lifestyle is really that of emphasizing the prevention of ill health and the ongoing procreation of mankind.

The concept of acid and alkaline balance is universal to all people, regardless of gender or ethnic origin. After the metabolism of food is complete, most mixed diets contain a surplus of acid-forming mineral elements that must be continually buffered to maintain acid-alkaline balance. But as cells are unable to rid themselves of these wastes, they become deposited first in the connective tissues, and then the organs or the body. These acids constantly eat away body tissues and interrupt the functions of the cells and organs.

Viruses, germs, bacteria and parasites thrive in an acid environment. A daily balance of nutritional foods should be a combination of a high intake of vegetable servings and fruits (organic, if obtainable), organic grain products, herbal teas and quality servings of proteins in the form of organic meat and eggs, as well as dairy produce from organic sources. Man-produced food items and non-organic foodstuffs contain a high proportion of chemicals such as food additives and preservatives, as well as many chemicals used during the farming of the produce, which all turn into acid-forming elements bombarding our tissues and congesting our meridians. Likewise, while dairy produce contains many alkaline-forming minerals, commercially produced dairy products contain acid-forming minerals and chemicals that the body cannot utilize or eliminate.

If the earth element is off-balance, all cycles lose their patterns – sleeping, breathing, thought processes, body harmony and coordination. Signs of distress in the earth element manifest in nervousness, instability, disconnectedness and insecurity.

The Stomach Meridian

A yang meridian with a descending flow of energy running from the head to the foot. It receives Chi from the large intestine meridian and passes it on to the spleen meridian. The stomach meridian starts under the eye and curves up to the temple; it then continues down the body and ends on the top of the second toe (see figure 7).

The Nei Ching states:

'The stomach acts as the official of the public granaries and grants the five tastes[16] ... In the stomach, lower intestines, the three burners, the groin and the bladder, one can find the basic principle for the public granaries and the encampment of a regiment. These organs are called "vessels" and have the power of transforming the dregs and the sediment and cause the flavours to revolve so that they enter the vessels and leave them. These organs influence the lips and cause flesh around them to be of light colour; these organs are effective upon the flesh and the muscles. The flavour connected with these organs is sweet and the colour is yellow.'[17]

The functions and activities of the stomach and spleen are closely related. The stomach controls digestion – it receives nourishment, integrates it and brings it to fruition, and passes on the 'pure' food energy to be distributed by the spleen.[18] The spleen then transforms it into the raw material for Chi and blood. If the stomach does not hold and digest food, the spleen cannot transform it and transport its essence. They are interdependent meridians. The directions of the Chi activity complement each other – the spleen rules ascending and the stomach rules descending.[19]

According to Chinese philosophy the stomach is related to appetite, digestion and transport of food and fluids, but the partner meridian, the spleen/pancreas, is responsible for the ruling of food transport and energy consumption. The two meridians of the earth element work together more closely to stabilize the individual than any of the others. The earth element represents harmony and if there is no harmony in the stomach, spleen and pancreas, this will affect all the other organs.

The stomach is referred to as the 'sea of food and fluid' or 'sea of nourishment' as it governs digestion and is responsible for 'receiving' and 'ripening' ingested foods and fluids. Without the nourishing activities of the stomach, the other organs in the body could not function. The stomach is central physically and functionally; thus any problem in the stomach is quickly reflected in the other organs.

If this organ is out of balance, whatever is taken in, be it physical or psychic food, will not be utilized correctly. Energy depletion – lethargy, weakness and debilitation – are symptoms warning us that this function is impaired.

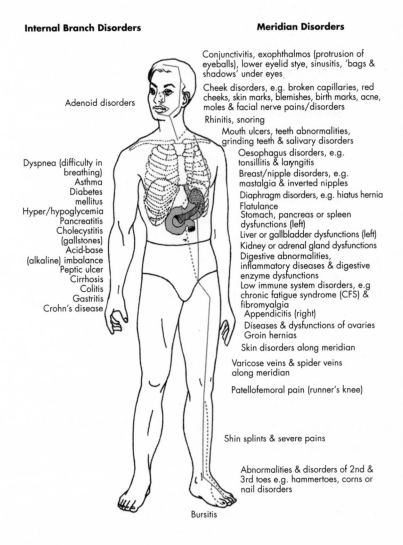

Internal Branch Disorders

Adenoid disorders

Dyspnea (difficulty in breathing)
Asthma
Diabetes mellitus
Hyper/hypoglycemia
Pancreatitis
Cholecystitis (gallstones)
Acid-base (alkaline) imbalance
Peptic ulcer
Cirrhosis
Colitis
Gastritis
Crohn's disease

Meridian Disorders

Conjunctivitis, exophthalmos (protrusion of eyeballs), lower eyelid stye, sinusitis, 'bags & shadows' under eyes

Cheek disorders, e.g. broken capillaries, red cheeks, skin marks, blemishes, birth marks, acne, moles & facial nerve pains/disorders

Rhinitis, snoring

Mouth ulcers, teeth abnormalities, grinding teeth & salivary disorders

Oesophagus disorders, e.g. tonsillitis & laryngitis

Breast/nipple disorders, e.g. mastalgia & inverted nipples

Diaphragm disorders, e.g. hiatus hernia

Flatulence

Stomach, pancreas or spleen dysfunctions (left)

Liver or gallbladder dysfunctions (left)

Kidney or adrenal gland dysfunctions

Digestive abnormalities, inflammatory diseases & digestive enzyme dysfunctions

Low immune system disorders, e.g chronic fatigue syndrome (CFS) & fibromyalgia

Appendicitis (right)

Diseases & dysfunctions of ovaries
Groin hernias

Skin disorders along meridian

Varicose veins & spider veins along meridian

Patellofemoral pain (runner's knee)

Shin splints & severe pains

Abnormalities & disorders of 2nd & 3rd toes e.g. hammertoes, corns or nail disorders

Bursitis

Fig. 7 Stomach meridian

Stomach meridian congestions

In this section, the symptoms are discussed in some depth as I believe disharmony in the stomach and therefore the pH (acid balance) to be the root cause of all diseases in the body. The quality of the food ingested goes hand in hand with the quality of life you enjoy. If the fuel is faulty, the functions of the organs will be faulty and disease will be the ultimate result. The stomach meridian is the only meridian that penetrates all the major body organs.

Beginning with the section of the meridian that runs through the face, many tactile observations will enable the practitioner to ask probing questions related to the patient's case history, thereby giving a more complete picture of their health profile. The meridian starts under the eye and conditions with the eyes such as conjunctivitis or lower eyelid stye are evidence that the stomach meridian is showing signs of weakness. Another interesting phenomenon related to this area is exophthalmos (protrusion of eyeballs). Most medical doctors relate this condition specifically to thyroid problems, especially goitre, but if you take note of the path of the partner meridian – the spleen/pancreas – you will notice that it has an internal branch that runs directly through the thyroid, linking disorders and malfunctions of the thyroid to the spleen/pancreas and its partner the stomach. Bags and dark shadows under the eyes are related to kidney disorders. The stomach meridian penetrates the kidneys: within the interrelationship of the Five Elements, the earth element controls or loses control of the water element, meaning that the acid/alkaline balance or imbalance of the stomach/spleen pancreas controls or loses control of the sodium/potassium balance in the cellular system that is ruled by the kidneys and bladder.

Sinus, sinus pain and hay fever (allergic rhinitis) also relate to the stomach meridian around the eye region. Broken capillaries or blemishes in the cheeks and red cheeks can be indicative of bronchial problems, spasms or lack of oxygen, and often a need for yawning or grasping for air. The stomach meridian passes through this area of the body as well, and the above is a sign of high acidity in the respiratory system making it difficult for the body to utilize the oxygen molecules efficiently. Snoring and adenoid disorders are also congestions to be found on the stomach meridian.

The meridian passes around the mouth area and problems here include sores in the corners of the mouth (which may be indicative of stomach or duodenal ulcers); mouth ulcers; problems with the teeth (specifically the molars), grinding teeth and salivary disorders such as drooling onto the pillow during the night. If babies have severe teething and dribbling problems it is advisable for mothers to look to the stomach as the cause, as teething problems are lessened if the stomach is well balanced. Teething problems often go hand in hand with nappy rash, which is caused by high uric acid content, so a decrease in acidic food intake would help solve the problem.

Endocrine imbalances are frequently described by the medical profession as the main reason for facial acne, especially in females where facial skin problems are regularly tied in with their menstrual cycle. However, one needs to take note that the stomach meridian runs through the ovaries, and the acne is rightly an expression of hormonal imbalances, though the unevenness of acid/alkaline and blood sugar problems will be accentuated during menstruation and/or ovulation and should be treated and understood as the main cause of the acne. Furthermore, the acne is evidence of dysfunctions of the ovaries and suppressing the acne by taking the contraceptive pill only adds to future problems, such as infertility. Further facial evidence of potential infertility due to dysfunctions of the ovaries can be observed by looking at the section between the nose and the upper lip. Increasingly, young females taking the oral contraceptive pills are developing signs of moustache or have developed vertical lines in the same area – this section is also on the stomach meridian.

Many people are born with birthmarks on the face. If they look into their family background, they may discover a history of stomach complaints or a tendency to eat food of high acid content. Frequently, during pregnancy expectant mothers will develop a craving for acidic foods such as oranges, pickles, sweets and chocolate, further upsetting the delicate acid/alkaline balance of the stomach.

Most oesophageal (throat) disorders such as tonsillitis and laryngitis, as well as the constant need to clear one's throat, can be related to the stomach meridian as it passes through this area. On the foot, in the reflex for the oesophagus, a callus build-up or a long, deep skin groove confirms a weakness in the area. Furthermore, plantar warts (verrucas) can be found on weak reflexes and therefore on the oesophagus reflex as well. The wart will not disappear even with radical treatments until the underlying cause has been dealt with – if found on reflexes relating to the organs and meridians of the earth element, the acid/alkaline, as well as blood sugar imbalances have to be adjusted before the warts will disappear.

From the throat, the meridian continues into the bronchial area, so imbalances here can result in lung/bronchial complaints such as bronchial spasm, emphysema, asthma, tight chest and mucus build-up. A large callus build-up on the ball of the foot, representing the lung reflexes, indicates a weak chest.

The meridian then runs through the nipple, and in women one will see complaints related to the menstrual cycle including ovulation, such as sore breasts, inverted nipples, fibroids or cysts in the breasts. In fact, there are four meridians that pass through the breast, so if a cyst were the problem, the exact position would have to be located in order to define the meridian on which the cyst is situated.

Did you know? - Breast cancer

Breast cancer can largely be avoided by learning to recognize the early warning signs within the meridians and the Five Elements. In TCM, congestions in the meridian system are assessed as the root cause of breast cancer, relating each section of the breast to a particular meridian, rather than emphasizing the breast itself. The incidence of breast cancer is on the increase and statistics claim that one in eight women will develop breast cancer in her lifetime. In the Western approach, there are no known definitive causes, but likely risk factors are emerging in research, including food items and stimulants (such as animal fat, cigarettes and high alcohol consumption). Pesticides used in the production of vegetables, fruits and animal feed are also being researched. These mimic the oestrogen in the body causing many signs of hormonal imbalances. Lately, debates on hormone replacement therapy (HRT) that women are now commonly prescribed in the early stages of menopause, seem to indicate a double risk of developing breast cancer. Recognizing the various small congestions along the meridians is the simplest form of warning to take action and responsibility towards a change in lifestyle and therefore a prevention of breast cancer.

Below the breasts the meridian passes through the diaphragm, accordingly problems here, for example hiatus hernia, could be indicative of stomach disorders. The meridian runs through the liver and gall bladder on the right side of the body, subsequently dysfunctions of these organs may be caused by the stomach, such as cholecystitis (gallstones), while on the left side of the body, the meridian runs through the stomach, spleen, pancreas and duodenum. Problems such as ulcers, acid

regurgitation, indigestion, blood sugar imbalance and appetite problems can be tied in here. When conditions become more serious and
chronic, the disorders will manifest on the internal section of the
meridian that runs mostly parallel with the meridian itself. Dyspnea
(difficulty in breathing), asthma, diabetes mellitus, hyper/hypogly-
caemia, as well as acid-base (alkaline) imbalances are some of the
possible disorders when conditions become serious. Furthermore, peptic ulcer, cirrhosis, colitis, gastritis and Crohn's disease can be added to
the list.

The meridian has a slight curve before entering the adrenals and kidneys on both sides. An imbalance in the adrenals and kidneys can often
be linked to allergic problems, blood pressure disorders, bladder or kidney infections, kidney stones and oedema. Again, the stomach meridian
penetrates these organs and can be traced as the cause.

As the meridian descends, it enters the large and small intestines,
affecting the digestion and this can be related to problems such as constipation, diarrhoea, diverticulitis and colic, as well as inflammatory
diseases in the digestive tract. Many of these congestions lead to low
immune system disorders such as chronic fatigue syndrome (CFS) and
fibromyalgia.

Further down, the meridian runs through the appendix (right side) and
ovaries, linking it to problems such as appendicitis, ovarian cysts, menstrual cycle complaints, infertility and blocked Fallopian tubes. In the
groin region, hernias often occur on the stomach meridian.

The meridian then runs down the thighs linking the stomach meridian
to thigh complaints, varicose veins and broken capillaries. Along the
path of the meridian, skin problems such as psoriasis, eczema and moles
can occur. When the meridian reaches the knees, careful note must be
taken of exactly where the problem is – six meridians run through the
knees at different points. The knee pain associated with the stomach

meridian is patellofemoral pain (runner's knee) and the partner meridian will have an effect on the medial aspect of patella; lower in the leg there may be associated disorders of the shin.

In the foot, the meridian runs along the dorsal area and ends in the second toe, as well as internally on the third toe. Problems may be expressed in pains or problems such as toe nailing fungus, corns, bent or malformed toes – hammertoes and the like. If the second toe is longer than the big toe, this can indicate a genetic weakness in the stomach meridian. This does not necessarily mean the person will have problems in the stomach area. If their lifestyle is healthy, it is unlikely, but if not, they would be more prone than others to imbalances in the stomach and its meridian. Some family members might suffer from arthritic conditions or sore joints and others might have ulcers and digestive problems. Finally, problems with the muscles related to the stomach – the neck and chest muscles – could be caused by excess acidity in the stomach.

Internal branch congestions

Adenoid disorders, dyspnea (difficulty in breathing), asthma, diabetes mellitus, hyper/hypoglycaemia, pancreatitis, cholecystitis (gallstones), acid-base (alkaline) imbalance, peptic ulcer, cirrhosis, colitis, gastritis and Crohn's disease.

Did you know? – Super sick from fast food

Recently, Morgan Spurlock made a documentary film in the USA to show what would happen to his body if he lived solely on a diet of junk food. At the beginning of the documentary, the 33-year-old Morgan is the picture of health and happiness as he embarks on his takeaway challenge.

Within days, however, his new diet takes its toll. Little wonder – he is gobbling an astonishing 27300 kilojoules a day (a healthy intake is 10500 for men and 8400 for women). In the 30 days he gains more than 11 kg. His blood pressure has shot up, his cholesterol level has soared and he has lost his sex drive. He was urged by doctors to stop or he would die. However, he argued he was not taking drugs or boozing heavily; he was doing what millions around the world do every day – pigging out on greasy fast food.

Dr Daryl Isaacs, one of the three experts hired to monitor Morgan's health, was stunned by his deterioration. Even worse, a test showed the impact on his internal organs. The liver test was the most shocking of all – it became very abnormal.

Muscles associated with the stomach meridian

PECTORALIS MAJOR (CLAVICULAR)
This chest muscle helps turn the arm in at the shoulder. Treating the reflexes for this muscle affects both the stomach and the emotional centres within the brain.[20]

LEVATOR SCAPULAE
These muscles in the back of the shoulders and neck are often found to be weak, causing the neck to twist with the head staying level. If there is persistent tension in this muscle, chiropractic adjustment of the neck may be necessary.[21]

NECK MUSCLES
These muscles are the anterior neck flexors in the front and sides of the neck. They can easily be affected by whiplash injuries, making it diffi-

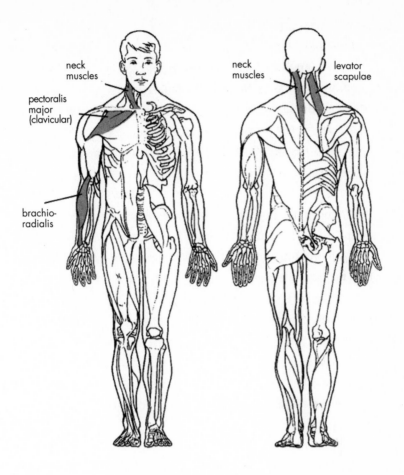

Fig. 8 Muscles associated with the stomach

cult to lift or turn the head. They are normally not quite as strong as the muscles in the back of the neck. If the muscles in the front become weak, the neck forms a C curve causing the head to balance improperly on the spine. This can be the source of headaches and shoulder tension.

BRACHIORADIALIS

This muscle flexes the elbow and helps turn the wrist. A weakness of this muscle may make it difficult to get the arm up and behind the back.[22]

Spleen/Pancreas Meridian

The spleen/pancreas meridian has an ascending (yin) flow of energy running from the foot to the chest. It obtains its energy from the stomach meridian and passes it on to the heart meridian. The spleen/pancreas meridian starts in the centre of the back of the big toe, ascends up the leg, through the body, and ends on one side of the breast under the armpit (see figure 9).

The Nei Ching states that: 'The spleen rules transformation and transportation.'[23] It is the crucial link in the process by which food is transformed into Chi and blood. If this process of food transformation is not activated, nourishment and Chi are not available for important body functions. If the transformative and transporting functions of the spleen are harmonious, Chi and blood can be abundant and digestive powers strong. If the spleen is in disharmony, the whole body or some part of it may develop deficient Chi or deficient blood.[24] Physiologically, the pancreas has considerable control over the body's nourishment, since its secretions help digest all the main constituents of food – proteins, fats and starch.

According to the Chinese, 'The spleen governs the blood' – it helps create blood and keeps it flowing in its proper paths. It is therefore associated with blood-excreting problems and it influences menstruation. The spleen also breaks down spent red blood cells and forms antibodies which neutralize poisonous bacteria, thus influencing immunity to infection. Chi and blood are transported to the muscles and flesh by the spleen via the circulatory system, therefore these too depend on the power of the spleen. The mouth and lips are closely related to the spleen. If the spleen is weak, the mouth will be insensitive to taste and the lips pale.[25]

Internal Branch Disorders   **Meridian Disorders**

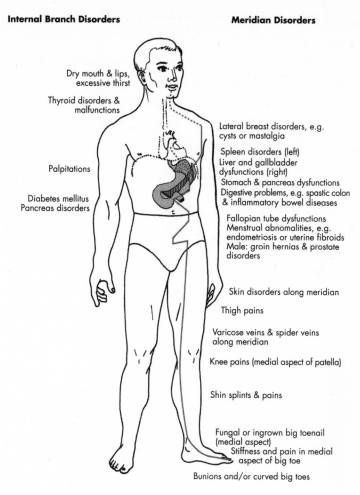

Dry mouth & lips,
excessive thirst

Thyroid disorders &
malfunctions

Lateral breast disorders, e.g.
cysts or mastalgia

Spleen disorders (left)
Liver and gallbladder
dysfunctions (right)
Stomach & pancreas dysfunctions
Digestive problems, e.g. spastic colon
& inflammatory bowel diseases

Palpitations

Diabetes mellitus
Pancreas disorders

Fallopian tube dysfunctions
Menstrual abnomalities, e.g.
endometriosis or uterine fibroids
Male: groin hernias & prostate
disorders

Skin disorders along meridian

Thigh pains

Varicose veins & spider veins
along meridian

Knee pains (medial aspect of patella)

Shin splints & pains

Fungal or ingrown big toenail
(medial aspect)
Stiffness and pain in medial
aspect of big toe

Bunions and/or curved big toes

Fig. 9 Spleen/pancreas meridian

Spleen/pancreas meridian congestions

The medial side of the big toenail relates to the spleen meridian, so stiffness, fungus or ingrown toenails here are indicative of problems of the spleen/pancreas meridian. As a reflexologist, take note of the condition of the big toe. If it curves inward – the beginning of the formation of bunions – this too indicates problems with this meridian and often the possibility would need to be ascertained of needs for stimulants, such as caffeine from tea and coffee, sweets, soft drinks, alcohol and cigarettes, or even too many fruits, carbohydrates or proteins.

Bunions occur on the spleen/pancreas meridian and the thyroid reflex – a section of the spleen/pancreas meridian runs through the thyroid. Tactile indicators of imbalances on the thyroid reflexes are often seen as a deep skin groove or a callus just below the phalanx and along the phalanx – the metatarsal joint. Many patients with bunions or even bursitis will often confirm a strong need for stimulants, as well as a strong need for being wanted and loved. Patients who have had their bunions removed time and again confirm a thyroid imbalance and the need for thyroid medication, and, vice versa, patients who have been taking thyroid medications for years frequently develop bunions later. Typically, a patient with bunions experiencing a stress situation will often release their emotional upsets by eating more stimulants. Either situation should be treated as a blood sugar condition and not necessarily symptomatic of bunions or even a thyroid complaint.

The meridian continues through the shin and the knee (medial aspect of the patella). Evidence of varicose veins and vein spiders, as well as skin disorders, will often be found on this meridian. Thigh pains, groin pains, hernias, and pelvic complaints in males such as prostate disorders. In females, menstrual abnormalities such as endometriosis or uterine fibroids often resulting in hysterectomies or infertility, and Fallopian tube dysfunctions that can lead to further infertility are related to the spleen/pancreas meridian and therefore to the unevenness of blood sugar balances.

As this meridian continues through the digestive area, problems include abdominal pain and distension related to spastic colon and inflammatory bowel diseases. Liver and gall bladder dysfunctions manifest on the right side of the body and spleen disorders on the left side of the body; also lateral breast disorders – lumps and cysts – and sensitivity and swelling prior to menstruation or ovulation. Again, it is important to look beyond the breast problem and instead relate to the meridian in question and take action on lifestyle changes (see the stomach meridian section, pages 89–99).

Did you know? – Infertility

Infertility in the developed world is on the increase, and is a problem for one in six couples, the male partner being responsible for half of the cases. Many young couples, when planning their children, have problems falling pregnant using the natural approach. Some researches are blaming electromagnetic waves from household appliances and telecommunications equipment, heavy smoking and liquor consumption, chemicals found in food and household products and the environment, and plastics in our food packaging.

In 1994, concern was expressed after a study revealed that men who eat organically grown food might be nearly twice as fertile as those who do not. Even the animal kingdom is showing evidence of concern. Industrial pollution is causing many of our sea animals around the world to show indication of sex changes and damage to the reproductive organs.

Female infertilities related to the stomach meridian

These can be understood and treated as acid/alkaline imbalances:

POLYCYSTIC OVARY SYNDROME (PCO)
A condition where the egg matures in the ovary but is not released into the Fallopian tube for fertilization. The ovaries produce high amounts

of male hormones, especially testosterone. At the onset of problems, many young females show signs of acne (also a symptom on the stomach meridian) along the jaw line of the face often being advised to take the contraceptive pill – suppressing all the symptoms but not dealing with the underlying cause.

Female infertilities relating to the spleen/pancreas meridian

These can be understood and treated as blood sugar imbalances:

UTERINE FIBROIDS
These are tumours of muscle tissue that imbed on the uterus wall. These fibroids can cause symptoms such as heavy bleeding, anaemia and bleeding between cycles. Oestrogen seems to stimulate their growth.

ENDOMETRIAL POLYPS
Smooth, tube-like growths, which may develop from the mucous membrane in any part of the body, including the uterus. They cause infertility and heavy menstruation if they grow in the corpus of the uterus.

FALLOPIAN TUBE DYSFUNCTION
This is often caused by blockages resulting from chronic inflammation in the tubes. Damage to the Fallopian tubes can prevent contact between the follicle (egg) and sperm, causing infertility.

ENDOMETRIOSIS
A condition where tissues of uterine lining migrate out of the uterus and implant in other abdominal tissues. Every month, when oestrogen causes the lining of the uterus to thicken, these cells expand and bleed. They cannot be released and result in cysts. It can be the basis for intense menstrual cramps and is very often a cause of infertility. There is no single symptom to let you know you have endometriosis, but pain is the most common one.

Infertilities relating to the liver meridian – female and males

These can be understood and treated as chemical stress to the liver through lifestyles:

CANDIDOSIS

Fungal yeast infection caused by Candida albicans is a common and normal inhabitant of the mucosal tissues, such as the mouth and vagina. However, the yeast can overgrow and produce an inflamed rash on the skin surfaces. Often the cause is unevenness in the Ph balance of the vagina making it a hostile environment for sperm. The acidity in the vagina, together with the yeast infection, rapidly immobilizes sperm. Many females with an infection will be prescribed antibiotics that will further place stress on the liver and therefore the liver meridian.

LOW SPERM COUNT/ABSENCE OF SPERM

This is the most common cause of infertility in men. Optimum sperm count for fertilization is around 100m per ml. A count below 20m officially constitutes reduced fertility and therefore a reduced chance of fathering a child. In addition, increasingly sperm have been observed to have deformed heads and kinked tails, and a growing proportion does not even swim towards the egg.

IMPOTENCE

Also known as erectile dysfunction, this is becoming common across the whole range of age groups and is often blamed on stress – rather than taking a closer look at congestions along the liver meridian and the lifestyle pattern of the men. Some research links depression to sexual dysfunctions, so again a close look to the internal part of the liver meridian is necessary.

SEXUALLY TRANSMITTED DISEASES

STDs such as herpes and gonorrhoea are known to reduce fertility.

Internal branch disorders

Dry mouth and lips and excessive thirst, thyroid disorders and malfunctions. Palpitations and diabetes mellitus, as well as pancreas disorders.

Did you know? – Diabetes

There is a widely understood connection between a strong thirst and dry mouth and potential diabetes. If asked what a doctor is going to check if one suffers from strong thirst and dry mouth, most people would say the blood sugar levels.

Nowadays more and more people suffer from diabetes or low blood sugar. However, it is interesting to note that there is no scientific explanation for the connection between the pancreas as an organ and the mouth. Nevertheless, this observation was first noted by the Chinese more than 5,000 years ago, but noted as an internal deep problem (as with thyroid disorders). Many of the concerns of modern society today relate to weight gain and increased likelihood of becoming a diabetic. Yet, it is an understanding of the spleen/pancreas meridian and its partner, the stomach meridian, that has to be brought to bear and taken as a warning sign before the condition develops into diabetes. Any females with irregular, heavy or painful menstrual cycles are being forewarned through the meridian system of low Chi; similarly with sore, swollen breasts on the lateral sides, or simple signs such as bunions and sore knees or even an ingrown toenail.

Many people feel the sensation of palpitations when the blood sugar dives. Again a small internal branch of the spleen/pancreas meridian goes to the heart and, if the blood sugar is in a constant fluctuation and the subject is satisfying their hunger and need for sugar stabilization by having a cup of coffee/tea or bar of chocolate, rather than nutritionally correct food, this will only be increasing the likelihood of long-term problems of the heart. One of the major risks for any patient with diabetes is condition of the heart.

Muscles associated with the spleen/pancreas meridian

LATISSIMUS DORSI
This muscle pulls the arm down and helps keep the back straight. It is used in forceful arm movements, such as swimming, rowing, bowling, golf and baseball swings. Because of its relationship with the pancreas where insulin is produced, people with diabetes, insulinaemia, hypoglycaemia and other problems of sugar metabolism will show weakness in this muscle. There will be a high shoulder on the weak side.[26]

TRAPEZIUS
This is one of the muscles that move the shoulder blade. It can be involved in shoulder and arm problems.[27]

EXTENSOR POLLICIS LONGUS
If the muscles of both hands are weak and do not respond, there may be a fixation of the sacrum. This weakness sometimes leads to 'tennis elbow'. The wrist bones, especially the radius and ulna, are not held in a good position and strain on the elbow results. This syndrome is complicated and may require professional advice and treatment.[28]

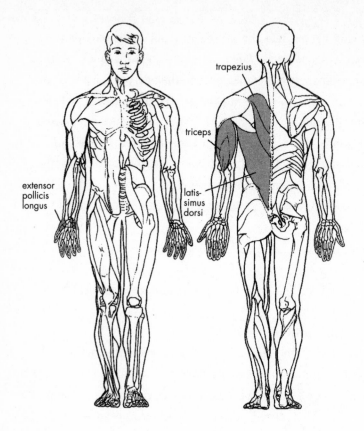

Fig. 10 Muscles associated with the spleen/pancreas

TRICEPS

These are situated in the back of the arm and help in straightening the elbow, working opposite the biceps. They can be affected by any of the problems of sugar metabolism which affect the latissimus dorsi.[29]

The behavioural patterns of the individual with earth element imbalances

THE SEASON: LATE SUMMER (INDIAN SUMMER)

In many of the translations of early Chinese literature, the earth element relates to a short season by some cultures named the 'Indian summer' – often a period where the weather suddenly seems warmer than expected. However, I feel that we should rather relate the earth element to the four times of seasonal changes and take note of the influences these days have on the weather around the globe. After the spring equinox (Northern hemisphere – 21 September; Southern hemisphere – 21 March) on which night's darkness equals the length of the day, nights become longer than days, until the winter solstice, the longest night and shortest day. (Northern hemisphere – 21 December; Southern hemisphere – 21 June). Close to the equinox, it is often at these times that hurricanes, major coastal storms and heavy rainfalls seem to take place, surprising people and nations. However, the havoc that appears in nature also happens within, and if our meridians are heavily congested and we are generally weak, this is often the time when more serious illness can start taking its toll. This again confirms the effect an imbalance in our earth element can have on our health.

THE EMOTION: SYMPATHY OR COMPASSION

The person who cannot receive sympathy, and the person who continually asks for sympathy, are both stuck and do not flow easily in and out of the emotion. This can be shown in attitude, posture, words and actions. A person might manufacture 'complaints' in order to gain sympathy from others, or others might show too much sympathy or lack any understanding. The 'I need chocolates/cigarettes/alcohol/love' is confirming an earth imbalance.

Note: It is important for therapists to take note and recognize their own imbalances – there is nothing worse than having a therapist who becomes the patient during a consultation. Often, unbeknown to the therapist, information given by the patient triggers the need for the therapist to 'share' their emotions with the patient. This can often lead to an inappropriate reversal of roles.

THE TIME OF DAY OF PEAK: STOMACH: 7–9 AM; SPLEEN/PANCREAS 9–11 AM

Breakfast is considered to be the most important meal of the day. Those who cannot eat breakfast are confirming an imbalance; likewise those who have a 'sugar dip' between 9 and 11 in the morning and a need for stimulants in order to feel 'alive' or energetic show further imbalances. Children who have eaten a sugar-loaded breakfast lose their concentration level by mid-morning and start eating their lunch or looking for sweets. They do not take in their lessons and will often be classified as hyperactive.

If we were to compare our body to a vehicle, it is likely that we do not treat it with the same respect and understanding that we give to our cars. We would never be able to drive our car on an empty tank, nor use the incorrect fuel. However, we expect to drive our body/vehicle without fuel; when we do not cope – as often happens – this will be put down to stress, rather than taking a look at our nutritional intake or the lack thereof. The state of our emotions is closely linked to our eating habits and our ability to process food, creating energy or Chi.

THE SOUND: SINGING

Singing, in this context, relates to the monotone non-melodious sound of speaking regardless of the words. It is like listening to a person without many different levels of sound waves but instead one continuous wave with many words. Listening to a speaker or newsreader reading a lot of information using in monotone way will 'sing' you to sleep!

We need to forgive 'boring' speakers but understand their imbalance and try to help. The sound from our voice box will change according to the balance or imbalance we are experiencing at that moment.

THE TISSUES: CONNECTIVE FATTY TISSUES (SOFT TISSUES)

These tissues are the covering of our body – the musculature that gives shape to each human being – and they go hand in hand with an understanding of 'flesh'. Sufferers from overweight have a shape that is larger and rounder while the flesh of those suffering from eating disorders loses shape and weight, making the body look undernourished and thin. In either case, this is confirmation that the earth element is out of balance and the patient needs to balance the acid/alkaline and blood sugar levels in order to bring about a balanced body weight and shape.

THE EXTERNAL PHYSICAL MANIFESTATIONS: FLESH

Patients who have pain in their flesh can often be very specific, knowing that they do not have pains in their bones, joints or muscles. Flesh refers to the musculature which gives each of us our shape. This is not the same as the skin or the muscles with which we mechanically move. The condition of the flesh shows whether there is a lack of nutrition in a person. However, the triceps muscles, situated in the back of the arm (see page 108), often become flabby, reflecting the state of their earth energy. Diseases such as chronic fatigue syndrome and fibromyalgia are typical of conditions of the flesh confirming the earth element and therefore the stomach and spleen/pancreas to be the underlying cause for their condition. Becoming 'blue bruised' easily or feeling pain when being hugged is a sign that is flesh is lacking nutrition.

THE SENSE ORGAN: MOUTH, LIPS

Our nourishment comes into our bodies through our mouths, and we exhale carbon dioxide. Signs of imbalance are evident when we use our mouth to take in our breath, rather than using our nose. Lips may be sore, swollen, cracked and have herpes (cold sores). The person who always has to use a lip balm to lessen dryness of the lips is reflecting an imbalance. Small children and babies that put everything they come into contact with into their mouths show evidence of lacking nourishment or the ability to process the food they are given. Mouth ulcers and sore gums further add to the list.

THE FLUID SECRETION: SALIVA

This is a close correspondence to the above. A person who complains of a lack of, or excess of, saliva confirms an imbalance of the earth element. Also, swallowing difficulties or drooling on to the pillow when sleeping and babies drooling when teething are signs of imbalances (see the spleen/pancreas meridian, page 100).

THE FLAVOUR: SWEET

There are many people who crave sweets and cannot 'live' without satisfying their needs throughout the day. However, the word 'sweet' that is used in all the translations surrounding the concept of the Five Elements does not cover the complete picture. We need to have an understanding of the ingredients, as well as food items that make the pancreas show stress and therefore produce more insulin than normal.

In addition, I would include all the foods and drinks that contain caffeine, such as coffee, tea and soft drinks, painkillers; also fermented foods such as alcohol, and processed and refined carbohydrates (for instance, modern wheat derivatives). Artificially ripened fruits are loaded with chemical sprays and high levels of chemical-loaded proteins, which all burden the function of the pancreas, as do all sugar-loaded sweets and foods. All of these foods, when used to satisfy cravings, show evidence of loss of control over the function of the pancreas.

THE SMELL: FRAGRANT

Although described as fragrant, the smell associated with an earth imbalance would more accurately be described as cloying or sickening-sweet. The smells emanating from a sick person are not always pleasant and are difficult to describe in words unless one has had the experience of them directly. The smell stemming from an imbalanced earth element is an unpleasant fragrance akin to the smell of flesh burning. It is not the scorch, but a sweetness that is most overwhelming. Patients who have suffered many years from diabetes and have lost control might experience this smell emanating from their mouth saliva. Even for those who have been consuming too much alcohol and sweet foods have this mouth odour, showing evidence that they are stressing the pancreas.

THE CLIMATE: DAMPNESS OR HUMIDITY

Weather has always affected the lives of human beings and has often been blamed for ill health. Most people living in a particular climate adjust to it and when they go to a different climate, they can experience a benefit or trauma to their health. A person who becomes ill or feels strong discomfort in humidity or, vice versa, a person who loves and only feels good in humidity are both confirming an imbalance in the earth element.

THE COLOUR: YELLOW

The Nei Ching states: 'when their colour is yellow like that of oranges they are without life'. The subtle hue of yellow emanating from the face tells us the condition of the earth element, as does a particular affinity or aversion to the yellow colour. One of my patients, many years ago, married a diabetic widower who had three children. It was a major adjustment in her life and she found it difficult to cater for them all with regards to meals, and she started having a 'love and hate' affair with the kitchen. She subconsciously expressed her needs for sympathy and compassion by decorating her kitchen in yellow. All her utensils were yellow, the walls and her curtains. Another patient suffering from infertility (the earth element) made a baby room ready with yellow colours as dominant.

THE FIRE ELEMENT

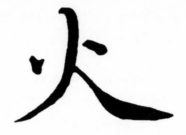

Fig. 11 Fire element

The element fire is seen as providing the energy governing the heart and small intestine. In addition, there are two other systems linked to the fire element, namely circulation/pericardium, which protects and regulates the blood flow, heat and nourishment throughout the body; the other system is termed the 'three heater', 'triple warmer' or 'three burners' and it acts to maintain proper temperature and warmth in the three cavities – respiration, digestion and elimination. In many Western translations, the three heater is described as the endocrine meridian as each of the three cavities also relates to hormonal glands and the functions thereof. Fire is light and warmth and its function in the body is not only to maintain heat but also to give warmth to others. The fire reflects the zest for life, the spark and vitality in body and mind. To be on fire is to be full of excitement about life. The fire imitates the quality of the food that has become Chi in the body; excess or lack of this can be expressed by many symptoms expressed, such as hot painful joints, fever, hot flushes, inflammations, heart burn and digestive problems, sexual coldness, lack of emotional warmth to other human beings (even those who are close), poor circulation of the blood that makes the extremities very cold, varicose veins and haemorrhoids. The two fire functions, circulation and heating, are important to the overall harmony of the body. As the Nei Ching states:

'If people pay attention to the five flavours and blend them well, their bones will remain straight, their muscles will remain tender and young, breath and blood will circulate freely, the pores will be in fine texture, and consequently breath and bones be filled with the essence of life.'

The Heart Meridian

The heart meridian has a descending (yin) flow of energy running from the chest to the hand. It gets its Chi from the spleen/pancreas meridian and in turn passes it on to the small intestine meridian. The heart meridian starts in the armpit and ends on the back of the little finger, towards the ring finger (see figure 12). The Nei Ching states:

> *'The heart is like the minister of the monarch who excels through insight and understanding*[30].... *The heart is the root of life and causes the versatility of the spiritual faculties. The heart influences the face and fills the pulse with blood.'*[31]

The heart and small intestine meridians are coupled. The Nei Ching explains their relationship:

> *'The heart controls the blood and unites with the small intestine. If the heart becomes heated, the heat will converge in the small intestine, producing blood in the urine.'*[32]

The classics also say:

> *'The heart rules the blood and blood vessels. Thus it regulates the blood flow, so when the heart is functioning properly, the blood flows smoothly. Therefore the heart, blood and blood vessels are united by their common activity. If the heart is strong, the body will be healthy and the emotions orderly; if it is weak, all the other meridians will be disturbed.'*[33]

It is also said that the heart rules the spirit. When the heart's blood and Chi are harmonious, spirit is nourished and the individual responds appropriately to the environment. If this is impaired, symptoms like insomnia, excessive dreaming, forgetfulness, hysteria, irrational behaviour, insanity and delirium may manifest.[34]

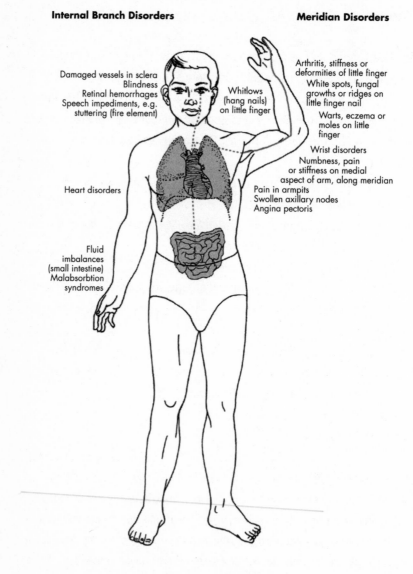

Internal Branch Disorders

Damaged vessels in sclera
Blindness
Retinal hemorrhages
Speech impediments, e.g.
stuttering (fire element)

Heart disorders

Fluid
imbalances
(small intestine)
Malabsorbtion
syndromes

Meridian Disorders

Whitlows
(hang nails)
on little finger

Arthritis, stiffness or
deformities of little finger
White spots, fungal
growths or ridges on
little finger nail

Warts, eczema or
moles on little
finger

Wrist disorders
Numbness, pain
or stiffness on medial
aspect of arm, along meridian
Pain in armpits
Swollen axillary nodes
Angina pectoris

Fig. 12 Heart meridian

Heart meridian congestions

Angina pectoris, pain in the armpits, swollen auxiliary nodes, numbness, pain or stiffness on medial aspect of arm along meridian. Wrist disorders, warts, eczema or moles on little fingers, white spots, fungal growths or ridges on little finger nails, as well as whitlows (hangnails on little fingers). Arthritis, stiffness or deformities of little finger.

Internal branch congestions

Damaged vessels in sclera, blindness and retinal hemorrhages, speech impediments (such as stuttering), heart disorders, fluid imbalances (small intestine) and malabsorption syndromes.

Muscle associated with the heart meridian

SUBSCAPULARIS
This muscle cannot be seen or felt because it is behind the scapula (shoulder blade). It allows the shoulder blade to glide over the rib cage and rotates the arm backwards, drawing the arm in when it is raised above the shoulder.[35]

The Small Intestine Meridian

The small intestine meridian has an ascending (yang) flow of energy running from the hand to the head. It receives its Chi from the heart meridian and passes it on to the bladder meridian. The small intestine meridian begins on the outside of the tip of the little finger and passes upward along the posterior aspect of the forearm. It circles behind the shoulder, then ascends along the side of the neck to the cheek and outer corner of the eye before entering the ear (see figure 14).

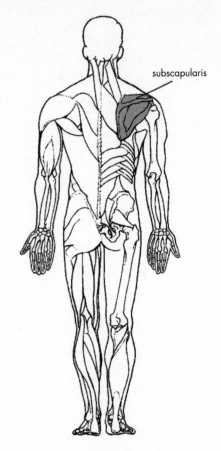

subscapularis

Fig. 13 Muscles associated with the heart

'The small intestines are like officials who are entrusted with riches and they create changes of the physical substance', says the Nei Ching.[36] The small intestine rules the separation of the 'pure' and the 'impure'. It contains the process of separation and absorption begun in the stomach. The functioning of the large intestine is influenced, both directly and indirectly, by the small intestine. In addition to passing solid residue on to the large intestine, the small intestine also controls the proportion of liquid to solid matter in the faeces, reabsorbing some liquids for the body's use and passing on the rest to be eliminated.[37]

The sorting out process – keeping that which has nutritional value and passing on waste to where it can be removed – happens on all levels of experience, both physiological and psychological; for example, sorting out the rubbish from that which is useful in terms of ideas, emotions and thoughts. If this sorting out function is not operating efficiently, symptoms that express this confusion may arise – hearing difficulties, the inability to sort out sounds from each other, and digestion problems resulting from poor sorting. Thus the flow relates not only to the assimilation of foodstuffs but also to the assimilation of experience, feelings and ideas for spiritual nourishment.

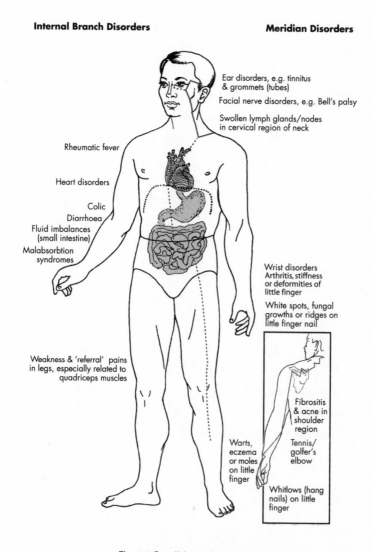

Internal Branch Disorders

Meridian Disorders

Ear disorders, e.g. tinnitus & grommets (tubes)

Facial nerve disorders, e.g. Bell's palsy

Swollen lymph glands/nodes in cervical region of neck

Rheumatic fever

Heart disorders

Colic

Diarrhoea

Fluid imbalances (small intestine)

Malabsorbtion syndromes

Wrist disorders Arthritis, stiffness or deformities of little finger

White spots, fungal growths or ridges on little finger nail

Weakness & 'referral' pains in legs, especially related to quadriceps muscles

Fibrositis & acne in shoulder region

Warts, eczema or moles on little finger

Tennis/ golfer's elbow

Whitlows (hang nails) on little finger

Fig. 14 Small intestine meridian

Small intestine meridian congestions

Arthritis, stiffness or deformities of little finger, white spots, fungal or ridges on the nail; whitlows (hang nails), warts, eczema or moles on little finger. Wrist disorders, tennis/golfer's elbow and fibrositis and acne in shoulder region. Swollen lymph glands/nodes in cervical region of neck, facial nerve disorders (such as Bell's palsy) and ear disorders (such as tinnitus).

Did you know? – Babies and colic

When a child is born, there are often complications during the birth process and the doctor or midwife may find it necessary to use forceps to guide the head through the birth canal; alternatively, strong finger grips in the same area may be used. The small intestine meridian runs on the head section exactly where the forceps or fingers are usually placed. This exerts undue pressure on this meridian, and this can be the cause of colic in young babies. The twisting action, which helps guide the baby through the birth canal, can also twist the spine and result in a slight structural spinal defect. To test whether the child has obstructions along the spine, hold the child upside down with a firm grasp around both ankles. If there are no spinal defects, the child's back will be straight, with the arms stretched out on either side. If the child hangs at a slight angle, this indicates a spinal defect, which requires the attention of a good chiropractor. Once the spine is corrected, colic problems should diminish.

Did you know? – Children and ear problems

Children in the younger age groups in developed societies often suffer from ear congestions which result in the need to have tubes (grommets) placed in their ears to alleviate the problem. Since the small intestine meridian ends in the ears, there will be a need to have a closer look at their nourishment. The quality of the 'baby formulas' used, as well as the overall quality of food or the lack thereof, should be taken into consideration. Are the children eating natural foods from a varied food chain, or are they living on man-made foodstuffs, lacking the essential building blocks necessary at early stages of development? Many busy parents buy their baby foods pre-cooked, believing it is nutritionally balanced. During pre-school age, toddlers are placed in a child-care system that often survives on creating large portions of non-expensive foods and drinks. Consequently, the child develops a blood sugar imbalance and finds it difficult to relate to 'normal' foods and instead continues to crave sugar-loaded artificial foodstuffs.

Internal branch disorders

Rheumatic fever, heart disorders, colic and diarrhoea; fluid imbalances (small intestine), malabsorption syndromes and weakness and 'referral' pains in legs, especially related to quadriceps muscles.

Muscles associated with the small intestine meridian

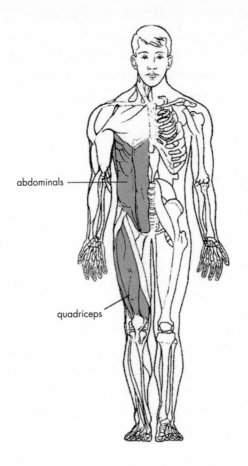

abdominals

quadriceps

Fig. 15 Muscles associated with the small intestine

QUADRICEPS

These straighten the knee and flex the thigh. Weakness will be evident when there is difficulty climbing stairs, getting up from or down to a seated position, picking the knee up, pain in the kneecap and other knee problems.[38]

ABDOMINALS

These muscles help keep the organs in place and bend the torso forwards and sideways. The rectus abdominis goes up and down the centre of the torso; the transverse abdominis goes underneath crosswise. They are associated with the duodenum, the first third of the small intestine, and are commonly involved in indigestion, stomach aches and breathing difficulties. Weakness of these muscles can result in a feeling of weakness or pain in the lower back. If weakness is only on one side, there may be some restriction of shoulder movement on the opposite side.[39]

The behavioural patterns of the individual with fire element imbalances

THE SEASON: SUMMER

Summer is the time when everything is in bloom and begins to bear fruit, everything flourishes and grows. From the foods grown in our gardens we should be eating and harvesting the highest Chi. This in turn will give us strong zest to carry us through autumn and winter. The Chinese considered the same process of fruition and ripening to happen with thought, experience, the body and emotions. If there is no bloom and the fruit does not grow, but withers and loses its life, a person will feel a general dissatisfaction in which nothing gets done. The person might feel cold within, longing for summer to feel warm or, if fire has lodged within and is trapped, summer heat might exacerbate the condition.

THE EMOTION: JOY AND HAPPINESS

We have many phrases in our language relating to the heart which we use without giving it a thought – feeling 'broken hearted', doing a job 'half-heartedly', being 'faint hearted' or, on the other hand, 'lion hearted' – all of which refer to joy, or lack of it, and our psychic strength surrounding the fire element. An excess of joy is as harmful as an excess of anger and the same goes for lack of joy. The desire for joy can become an impossible thirst causing something to give. Heart attacks are often a desperate attempt by the body and mind to alert us to a deficiency of the emotion joy. It is interesting to note that all four meridians belonging to the fire element have internal branches to the heart and that in the developed world more than 25% of people will die at an early age of heart-related conditions. Emotionally, the fire element relates to love, happiness, gentleness and forgiveness. The element stimulates both physical body warmth and psychological warmth in our relationships with others. Lack of concern and love for others, as well as lack of energy to love oneself, is indicative of an imbalance on the emotional plane. One may also find it very difficult to forgive.

THE TIME OF DAY OF PEAK: HEART 11AM–1PM; SMALL INTESTINE 1–3PM; CIRCULATION/PERICARDIUM 7PM–9PM; TRIPLE BURNER 9–11PM

The heart being the hard-working ruler of the body serves each cell in pumping some 3,000 gallons of blood per day to the neighbouring lungs, through which all blood must pass to obtain oxygen. Then the blood is returned to the heart, which pumps it out to the body, so all the parts can receive this nourishing breath of life.[40]

In order for the heart to daily do its job, the heart itself needs plenty of nourishing Chi from the food chain and the breath we take, and noon is the peak time for this process. However, if the Chi is insufficient and the heart does not receive enough, this may lead to a sudden tightness of the chest and the onslaught of a heart attack. Between 1–3pm is the peak time for the small intestine to be able to deliver and nourish our body with well-digested foods that have become Chi – especially following a wholesome breakfast. The opposite happens if no breakfast or an inappropriate meal has been taken and the body starts showing signs of being malnourished. The early and late evening is when the second round of feeling the fire emerges; however, if not enough fire is burning within the body, a feeling of being cold and lifeless with a lack of appetite for activity might surface, but if the rhythm and natural function are in order, the natural time to be in bed, and thus the natural time for love making, is between 9–11pm.

THE SOUND: LAUGHING

An absence of laughter or superficial laughter accompanies a fire imbalance; or a subtle hint of laughter in a person's voice even during the saddest conversation or a sound that is oftentimes a continuous giggle in an inappropriate situation confirms lack of fire. A never-ending jokester is the other side of a humourless, joyless person.

THE TISSUES: BLOOD VESSELS AND OUR PSYCHE

The temperature of the hands, feet and nose reveal the state of Chi within our circulation, as well as the general state of body relaxation. Labels such as hardening of the arteries, varicose veins, cold hands and feet are all symptoms confirming a lack of fire. Nervousness and apprehension create constriction of the blood vessels as part of the 'flight or fight' response to deal with stress and potential danger. Relaxation is important for the health, for keeping the rhythm of life and for our psyche to feel alive rather than lethargic and slow in action and thoughts.

THE EXTERNAL PHYSICAL MANIFESTATION: COMPLEXION

The complexion of a person reflects the fire; it is a description of the face texture, quality and skin. A good fire will show the presence of a glow and the feeling of a strong aura, whereas low fire will be expressed with facial dullness and a poor and aging quality of skin.

THE SENSE ORGAN: THE TONGUE

An expression used of people who talk non-stop is that they have 'verbal diarrhoea' or, conversely, that they are 'tongue-tied'. The tongue largely controls speech and many speech patterns such as stuttering and slurring or inability to find the right words give evidence of a weak fire element. Many young children in modern society are in need of speech therapy – however, the question of correct nourishment has to come into the equation. The tongue must be moist and pink; if it is red then the fire or heart may be too strong, which could lead to an inability to relax or slow down. If the tongue is pale, anaemia can be the problem.

THE FLUID SECRETION: PERSPIRATION

The Nei Ching states:

> 'If people do not perspire freely in the heat of summer, they will get intermittent fever in fall. If people perspire [only] partially, they contract a partial paralysis. When perspiration becomes visible and meets with humidity, there will be eruptions on the skin and a weakened condition.'

THE FLAVOUR: BITTER

An imbalance in the fire element is likely to give rise to a need for bitter flavours such as strong coffee, tea or dark chocolate (without sugar). Some will nibble on the charcoaled or burnt meat when barbecuing, or enjoy a burned slice of toast. A better way of satisfying the need for bitter flavour would be green leafy vegetables.

THE SMELL: SCORCHED, BURNT

Any major imbalance in the fire element can be smelled on a person's body. It is unmistakable once experienced, and in some cases overpowering. This is not body odour, but rather a distinct other scent. Considering that it is the element fire, it makes empirical sense that the smell would be a scorched, burnt odour.

THE CLIMATE: HEAT

A person who dislikes hot or even warm weather as they find it difficult to regulate their body temperature with perspiration (see 'Fluid Secretion' above), or loves it, as their fire within is burning on a low flame and the body is feeling cold is likely to be expressing an imbalance of the fire element.

THE COLOUR: RED

A red hue to the face or aspects of the face; red or white fingernails are evidence of an imbalance of the fire element. Other places to watch out for signs of imbalances are the palms of the hands and the body in general. A person whose body is reddish-purple, even on a warm summer day, is showing weak circulation (fire element). Loving or detesting red in a person's home and clothing points to imbalance.

THE WATER ELEMENT

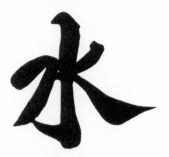

Fig. 16 Water element

By studying the element water, you can see the similarity between the human body and the planet Earth. In fact, seawater is almost identical to blood plasma and they both consist of 93–96% water with the remaining percentages of organic/inorganic compounds being very similar in composition. Water is the circulatory system of the Earth. Clouds, mountain snow, lakes, rivers, streams and the oceans are all part of this water circulation. Water is the essential medium of our body, through which all things pass. This fluid of life is important for functions throughout the body; the lymphatic flow, which helps to process and eliminate wastes and provides the ability to fight off infections and other foreign agents; and for the flow of urine, saliva, perspiration, tears, and sexual fluids.

Water must stay in motion; it has a rhythm, a cycle, which is ruled primarily by the movement and gravitational pull of the moon. The daily expansions and contractions of the oceans in the tides are like the breathing cycle of the Earth. The state of the water element in your body may reflect the state of your emotions. Like the planet, you can also have droughts and floods, stagnant pools and fresh flowing streams.

The Bladder Meridian

This meridian has a descending (yang) flow of energy running from the head to the foot. It receives its energy from the small intestine and passes it on to the kidney meridian. It is the longest meridian line in the body. The bladder meridian starts at the inner corner of the eye, continues over the crown of the head, down the back and legs, and ends on the outer edge of the back of the little toe (see figure 17).

'The groins and the bladder are like the magistrates of a region, they store the overflow and the fluid secretions which serve to regulate vaporization,' states the Nei Ching.[41]

The partnership of the kidney and bladder meridians is one of the most obvious. The function of the bladder is to receive and excrete urine produced in the kidneys from the final portion of turbid fluids transmitted from the lungs, small intestine and large intestine. It is therefore in charge of maintaining normal fluid levels in the body. It is not merely an excretory organ but is coupled with the function of the kidneys in helping to store the jing or vital essence (see 'kidney meridian' on page 136). The bladder is essential to life. If it is not functioning properly, the rest of the system is stressed and poisoned.[42]

The bladder meridian has a pronounced effect on the spinal cord and nerves, and is most effective in releasing tension along its path.

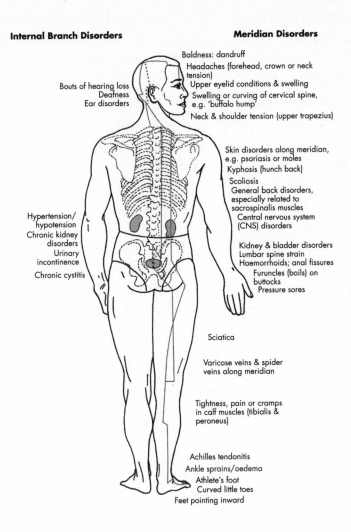

Internal Branch Disorders

Bouts of hearing loss
Deafness
Ear disorders

Hypertension/
hypotension
Chronic kidney
disorders
Urinary
incontinence

Chronic cystitis

Meridian Disorders

Baldness: dandruff
Headaches (forehead, crown or neck tension)
Upper eyelid conditions & swelling
Swelling or curving of cervical spine, e.g. 'buffalo hump'
Neck & shoulder tension (upper trapezius)

Skin disorders along meridian, e.g. psoriasis or moles
Kyphosis (hunch back)
Scoliosis
General back disorders, especially related to sacrospinalis muscles
Central nervous system (CNS) disorders

Kidney & bladder disorders
Lumbar spine strain
Haemorrhoids; anal fissures
Furuncles (boils) on buttocks
Pressure sores

Sciatica

Varicose veins & spider veins along meridian

Tightness, pain or cramps in calf muscles (tibialis & peroneus)

Achilles tendonitis
Ankle sprains/oedema
Athlete's foot
Curved little toes
Feet pointing inward

Fig. 17 Bladder meridian

Bladder meridian congestions

Most people acknowledge some of the congestions along the bladder meridian as health problems they suffer from, especially headaches (forehead and crown), as well as neck tension. Also, the combinations of neck and shoulder tension (upper trapezius) are normal pains that are accepted as stress related. Some blame their sitting or driving

positions and others to lifting heavy objects, leading to a visit to the chiropractor or a massage therapist to try and release their tensions.
However, we need to look at stress more closely. Does our lifestyle stress
the functions of our urinary system? Do we drink the wrong quality or
quantity of liquids? Many health advisors emphasize a need to drink lots
of water daily – without looking at the complete picture. The most
important aspect of our cellular system is keeping the fluid balance in
harmony; however, this does not necessarily mean drinking a large
quantity of liquids, but rather keeping the balance between the two
important minerals that keep the cells alive in their processes of daily
metabolizing inputs and outputs of nutritional foodstuffs. Inside the
cells there is potassium, and outside the cell walls there is sodium. By
eating plenty of natural products such as vegetables, fruits, herbs, nut,
seeds and legumes we support the balance of potassium and sodium
without having to drink extra liquid. Remember, a sign of thirst can be a
sign of blood sugar imbalance (see the 'Earth element', pages 87–92). The
eating of natural foods will also help prevent the dehydration of cells.

Did you know? – 'Buffalo hump'

The swelling or curving of the cervical spine known as 'buffalo hump' is an interesting condition. The area of the hump
is usually around cervical vertebra number 7, which is linked
through the nervous system to the function of the thyroid,
shoulder and elbow. The internal branch of the kidney
meridian (partner to the bladder meridian) passes through
the parathyroid that deals with our calcium absorption. It is
possible that we will be looking at the bladder and kidneys
for conditions relating to our bones, rather than in females
linking conditions to a hormonal imbalance. The Chinese
system indicates this.

Further congestions on the bladder meridian are upper eyelid conditions and swelling, baldness and dandruff. Skin problems along the meridian, such as psoriasis or moles, may be observed. Furthermore, the bladder meridian is the only meridian that covers the back of our body and therefore spinal and back disorders such as kyphosis (hunch back), scoliosis and general back disorders, especially related to sacrospinalis muscles can be related to a bladder/kidney imbalance, as well as lumbar spine strain. Problems with the central nervous system (CNS), as well as the organ functions of the kidneys and bladder; haemorrhoids, anal fissures and furuncles (boils) on buttocks, as well as pressure sores; sciatica pains, varicose veins and spider veins along the meridian, tightness, pain or cramps in calf muscles (tibialis and peroneus); Achilles tendonitis, ankle sprains/oedema, athlete's foot, curved little toes and feet pointing inward (pigeon toes) – a minor physical defect often found in young children is a tendency to walk with their feet turned inwards (this may be combined with a tendency to bedwetting) – are all problems along the bladder meridian. If the kidney/bladder reflexes are strengthened these problems will be rectified.

Did you know? – Bladder meridian and sexual function

In the ankle region it is interesting to find that the bladder meridian penetrates the sexual organ reflexes that are often sensitive to stimulation, but without necessarily any confirmation of problems or malfunction. When stimulating the reflex, we are also stimulating the bladder meridian, and the bladder and kidney meridians have an indirect connection to the function of the sexual organs. As well as having an effect on the sexual organ reflex, the uterus/prostate reflex also tends to be more sensitive because of an imbalanced kidney meridian, rather than having actual uterus/prostate problems.

The bladder meridian runs down the back next to the spinal cord. It will be observed that the reproductive organs receive their nerve supply from the sacrum. The lower back area is often massaged during childbirth to alleviate the pain experienced during this process. Many women also experience severe back pain during their menstrual cycle. In both instances, the reproductive system is very active at this time.

Internal branch congestions

Bouts of hearing loss and deafness, as well as ear disorders. Hypertension/hypotension, chronic kidney disorders, urinary incontinence and chronic cystitis.

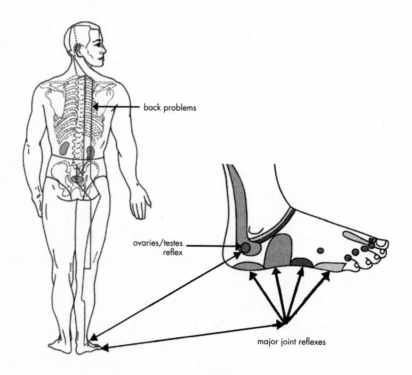

Fig. 18 Bladder meridian and sexual function

Muscles associated with the bladder meridian

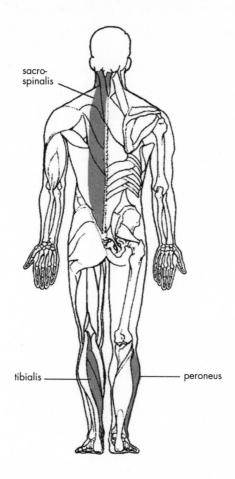

sacro-
spinalis

tibialis

peroneus

Fig. 19 Muscles associated with the bladder

PERONEUS

This is the lower leg muscle, which flexes the side of the foot upward and out. Weakness will cause the foot to turn in, especially in children, and can also be associated with ankle and foot problems.[43]

SACROSPINALIS

This is a group of several separate muscles along the backbone. It can be the cause of 19 different areas of pain and malfunction in the spine and is associated with problems of arthritis, rheumatism, bursitis, shoulder and elbow problems. Weakness on one side will cause a bending of the spine, which can become a serious problem if neglected. Weakness on both sides will create the posture seen on many skinny people: the abdominal muscles contracted, the head and hips forward and the spine pushed back. This muscle is closely associated with bladder problems and may also be affected by emotional strain.[44]

TIBIALIS ANTERIOR

This muscle flexes the foot in and upwards and is often found to be weak on both sides. Weakness can be associated with rectal fissures, and urethra and bladder problems.[45]

The Kidney Meridian

The kidney meridian has an ascending (yin) flow of energy running from the foot to the chest. It receives Chi from the bladder and passes it on to the pericardium meridian. The kidney meridian starts on the sole of the foot and ascends up the back of the leg. It emerges around the front of the lower thigh and ascends straight up the body to the breastbone (see figure 20). The Nei Ching states:

> 'The kidneys are like officials who do energetic work and they excel through their ability[46] ... The kidneys call to life that which is dormant and sealed up; they are the natural organ for storing away, and they are the place where the secretions are lodged. The kidneys influence the hair on the head and have an effect upon the bones.'[47]

> 'The kidneys store the Jing and rule birth, development and maturation. Jing is the substance – a vital essence – which is the source of life and individual development. It has the potential for development into yin and yang and therefore produces life. The body

and all the organs need Jing to survive, and because the kidneys
store Jing, they bestow this potential for life activity. They there-
fore have a special relationship with the other organs because the
yin and yang, or life activity, of each organ ultimately depends on
the yin and yang of the kidneys. Jing is the source of reproduction,
development and maturation, so all these processes are governed
by the kidneys. Reproductive energy is produced manifesting as
sperm and ova.' [48]

The kidneys regulate the amount of water in the body. Fluids are essential to life as it bathes the entire cellular system. The flow of fluids enables waste material to be collected and excreted in the form of urine. Enormous amounts of blood flow through the kidneys to be purified and broken down into nutritional components for the body. [49]

The kidneys rule the bones and produce marrow. As the teeth are related to hard connective tissues, the kidneys also rule them. There is a close relationship between the kidneys and the ears, and normal breathing also requires assistance from the kidneys. They also influence the adrenal glands and parathyroids, and have a close connection with the spinal column, as the kidney meridian ascends the spine to the skull. [50]

Kidney meridian congestions

Burning, sweating or painful soles of the feet; eczema or fungus on the soles of the feet; feet pointing outward and ankle sprains and oedema are all weaknesses around the foot and ankle that have to be understood as being weaknesses with the bladder and kidneys and the water element. The meridian follows the medial aspect of the calf and pains in this area; since the tibialis anterior muscle that is governed by the bladder is in the same area, this makes for strong connections to the bladder and kidneys. Dorsal knee pain is on the kidney meridian. Skin

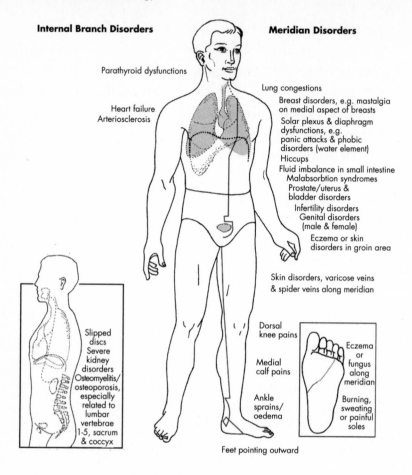

Internal Branch Disorders

Meridian Disorders

Parathyroid dysfunctions

Heart failure
Arteriosclerosis

Lung congestions
Breast disorders, e.g. mastalgia
on medial aspect of breasts
Solar plexus & diaphragm
dysfunctions, e.g.
panic attacks & phobic
disorders (water element)
Hiccups
Fluid imbalance in small intestine
Malabsorbtion syndromes
Prostate/uterus &
bladder disorders
Infertility disorders
Genital disorders
(male & female)
Eczema or skin
disorders in groin area

Skin disorders, varicose veins
& spider veins along meridian

Slipped
discs
Severe
kidney
disorders
Osteomyelitis/
osteoporosis,
especially
related to
lumbar
vertebrae
1-5, sacrum
& coccyx

Dorsal
knee pains

Medial
calf pains

Ankle
sprains/
oedema

Eczema
or
fungus
along
meridian

Burning,
sweating
or painful
soles

Feet pointing outward

Fig. 20 Kidney meridian

disorders and varicose veins and spider veins can often be traced along the pathway of the meridian, even eczema or skin disorders in the groin area are often traced to the kidney meridian; also genital, as well as infertility disorders; bladder, prostate and uterus disorders. The kidney meridian penetrates the small intestine and can be the underlying reason for malabsorption syndromes, as well as fluid imbalance in the small intestine. Lung congestions, solar plexus (where we feel the 'fight-or-flight' response triggered by adrenaline) and diaphragm dysfunction, such as panic attacks and phobia, as well as hiccups; breast disorders, such as mastalgia on medial aspect of breasts.

Internal branch congestions

Parathyroid dysfunctions, heart failure and arteriosclerosis in the upper section of the internal branch. Slipped discs and severe kidney disorders, as well as osteomyelitis and osteoporosis especially related to lumbar vertebrae 1–5, sacrum and coccyx.

Muscles associated with the kidney meridian

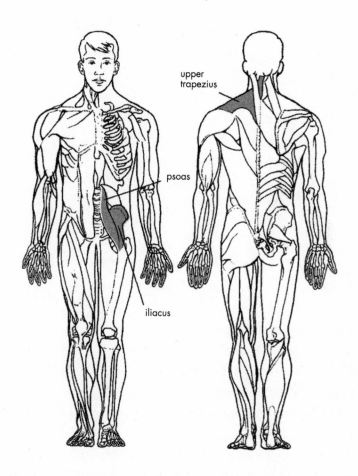

Fig. 21 Muscles associated with the kidney

PSOAS

This is part of the spine-flexing group and helps keep the lumbar curve in the spine. With weakness on both sides there will be a tendency for the lower back to flatten. Weakness on one side will cause the foot to turn in or make the hip low. Standing or walking with the ankles turned in will put a strain on the psoas and can cause recurring weakness if the foot problem is not corrected. Nagging low back pain, kidney disturbances and foot problems can be associated with psoas weakness.[51]

UPPER TRAPEZIUS

This muscle tilts the head back and pulls the shoulder blade up. This will weaken with any problems associated with the ears and eyes.[52]

ILIACUS

This muscle, if weak, may indicate a problem with the ileo-caecal valve, the muscular valve between the small and large intestines. If the muscles are weak, an extensive set of symptoms may develop including nausea, sudden low back pain, shoulder pain, headache, sudden thirst, dark circles under the eyes and pallor.[53]

The behavioural patterns of the individual with water element imbalances

THE SEASON: WINTER

December 21 (Northern hemisphere) and June 21 (Southern hemisphere) is the date of winter solstice, midwinter's day and the day with the longest night and shortest day. One needs to stay active in order to keep the body warm and the energy moving; however, it is also the time to get plenty of rest and eat good wholesome root vegetables. If there is an imbalance in the water element, this season can be difficult to cope with, symptoms become more pronounced and the cold settles deep into the bones.

THE EMOTION: FEAR AND PHOBIAS

If the Chi energy is flowing well, we can experience life like the flow of a river; if it is not flowing well, we experience life like a nightmare, feeling overwhelmed and sinking into despair. Fear and phobias can be either a cause or a consequence of a water imbalance. Taking into consideration the time zones of the day (see below), a mother might start showing fears in the afternoon – fears for her husband being on his way home from work, fears for herself being caught in the traffic – after having been 'perfectly' OK during the day, which gives evidence to the state of her water element, making her feel 'blue' and anxious.

THE TIME OF DAY OF PEAK: BLADDER 3–5PM; KIDNEY 5–7PM

An imbalance may make the person feel sleepy, droopy, irritable or anxious, as well as having a stronger need to urinate. Many young families with small children might find this a difficult time if, say, having to do the shopping with the children, helping with their schoolwork and generally coping with everyone's irritability. Others might feel the effect of their high or their low blood pressure to be more pronounced.

THE SOUND: GROANING (MOANING OR HUMMING)

The voice box of the 'irritable' children shopping with their mother might be heard throughout the store as being pervasive, so expressing their water element imbalance, especially in the late afternoon (see above). Your friend or mother might be on the phone in the late afternoon with a voice that continually moans and groans, even though her life is no more problem-ridden than average. The sound happens in spite of herself.

THE TISSUES: BONES, BONE MARROW, NAILS AND TEETH (HARD CONNECTIVE TISSUES)

Referring back to the internal section of the kidney meridian going through the parathyroid (see page 130), the link to the hard connective tissues becomes understandable. This includes all the bones: the skull, the extremities and the spine, as well as the teeth and the bone marrow.

Split, soft or peeling nails are evidence of imbalance. Expressions such as, 'I feel it in my bones' suggest a strong link to our emotional experiences and the water element.

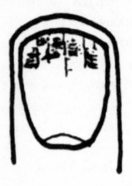 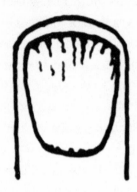

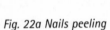

Fig. 22a Nails peeling   *Fig. 22b Nails split*

THE EXTERNAL PHYSICAL MANIFESTATION: HEAD HAIR

Assessing the condition and energy of a person's head hair – for instance, whether it is brittle, dry, broken or split; whether the person suffers from baldness, dandruff or lifeless thinning hair – all point to signs of lack of Chi in the water element (see pathway of the bladder meridian, fig 17).

THE SENSE ORGAN: EARS

Problems of hearing may reflect a water element disharmony (see pathway of the bladder meridian, figure 18). Fluid is part of the hearing process and is controlled by the water element. It is interesting to note that the shape of the ears and kidneys are similar, as is the human embryo. The embryo, and later the foetus, grow in the water medium, through which sounds travel to the developing ears. Bouts of deafness can be considered to show a bladder/kidney and water element disharmony.

THE FLUID SECRETION: SPITTLE

There are two distinct saliva secretions produced in the mouth – one we have spoken about with regard to the earth element (see page 93); the

other, spittle, is the saliva governed by the water element which bathes
our teeth. Our teeth are always wet, making it possible to speak without our lips sticking onto our teeth. However, apprehensive speakers are
often given a glass of water to help them not to feel dry in the mouth;
nervous speakers (see 'Fears and Phobias' above) frequently cannot
avoid using their tongue to lubricate their teeth. An elderly person with
chronic bladder or kidney infections might also experience dry teeth
and will use the tongue to alleviate the dryness.

THE FLAVOUR: SALTY

A person who use plenty of salt with their food before tasting it confirms
a disharmony in the water element, as does a person who finds difficulty eating food cooked with the slightest hint of salt. In Western medicine,
it is widely recognized that too much salt is a cause of water retention,
high blood pressure and kidney and heart trouble. The salt balance in our
body will stay in harmony through eating foodstuffs from natural food
chains that contain sodium, potassium, calcium and magnesium.

THE SMELL: PUTRID

This is a quite distinct and not easily described smell; it is more acrid
and putrefied than urine and, in the case of severe bladder and kidney
problems, the smell is quite strong – even a hint of this smell suggests
an imbalance in the water element.

THE CLIMATE: COLD

Anyone who suddenly feels cold may experience the need to urinate.
We cannot relax our body when feeling cold and many cannot fall
asleep if they have cold feet. Often, when feeling cold, we cross our
arms across our diaphragm and solar plexus and try to feel less tight in
our body. A person who has imbalances within the water element
brings on weaknesses when cold – yet others only feel healthier in the
cold season, also confirming an imbalance. The expression 'cold feet' is
often used when describing a person who becomes nervous or fearful
and opts out of a situation (see 'Emotion' above).

Did you know? – Maintaining the right temperature

During my many years as a therapist, I have often pointed to the importance of making sure our body temperature stays constant. In the northern latitudes where it is generally cold in the winter months, we were always taught to make sure that our feet were kept warn and dry with the correct footwear and socks, as well to wear a warm hat in winter. Moving to South Africa, where it is warm and often hot, in which climate my two sons were brought up, I noticed that small children were encouraged to take off their socks and shoes in order to play. When shopping with their mothers, young children would walk barefoot on the cold ceramic tiles in large air-conditioned stores.

We know the moment our body temperature rises by one to two degrees that we have a fever. However, it is less understood that lowering our temperature by a few degrees also makes our body vulnerable. The analogy I use is to compare our body temperature to that of leaving the car outside the garage at night. During the summer months, when day and night temperatures are similar, the car will be dry in the morning, whereas when the nights are much colder than the day, the car will be wet in the morning with dew or frost.

The moment our body cools down we create the same phenomena – those of condensation. Small children express the event by having streaming noses or urinating more frequently and some will have sneezing fits. And if they stay cold, the meridians will become congested with stagnant Chi and this will bring on fever.

The feet are directly linked to all the body organs through the science of reflexology, as well as six of the main meridians. The bladder and kidney meridians are both found in the little toes, with the kidney meridian also running across the sole of the feet. Keep your feet warm and many health problems might never become an issue.

THE COLOUR: BLUE

A person coming home from clothes shopping, who has a water element imbalance, might well add more blue clothing to a wardrobe that is already primarily blue. Similarly, it is likely that their beddings, curtains, carpet and ornaments will be blue. A blue hue to the face, especially around the eyes, shows even in Western medicine that the kidneys are under stress.

The Pericardium/Circulation Meridian

The pericardium meridian has a descending (yin) flow of energy running from the chest to the hand. It obtains its Chi from the kidney meridian, and passes it on to the triple burner meridian. The meridian starts next to the nipple and descends down the arm ending on the back of the middle finger, towards the ring finger (see figure 24).

It is said that diseases of the heart are borne by the pericardium. The pericardium is the outer protective shield of the heart – a loose fibrous sac, which encloses a slippery, lubricated membrane to prevent friction as the heart beats. Its role is to defend the heart from stress, shocks and other harmful influences. The West does not recognize this particular system as an organ and, technically, it is not. But the Chinese appreciated that an organ does not have to be in one piece to be effective, so they considered the whole vascular system to be an organ in itself. This system includes the arteries, veins and capillaries, which deal with the circulation of fluid in the body. The pericardium meridian is also known as the heart constrictor, heart circulation or circulation meridian. The pericardium and triple burner are partner meridians. Both have protective functions, and neither is an organ in the strict technical sense of the word. If the triple burner is imbalanced, the organs are deprived of proper nourishment and revolt against the heart. If the pericardium is weak, the heart will be vulnerable and the nourishing activities of the triple burner will be less effective.[54]

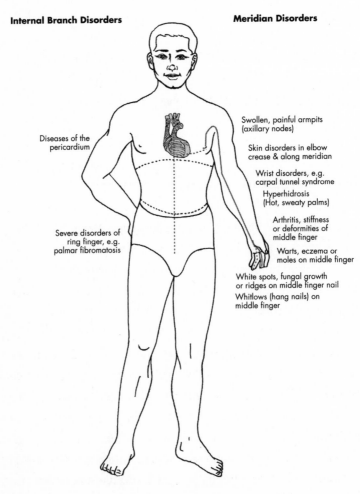

Internal Branch Disorders

Diseases of the pericardium

Severe disorders of ring finger, e.g. palmar fibromatosis

Meridian Disorders

Swollen, painful armpits (axillary nodes)

Skin disorders in elbow crease & along meridian

Wrist disorders, e.g. carpal tunnel syndrome

Hyperhidrosis (Hot, sweaty palms)

Arthritis, stiffness or deformities of middle finger

Warts, eczema or moles on middle finger

White spots, fungal growth or ridges on middle finger nail

Whitlows (hang nails) on middle finger

Fig. 23 Pericardium/circulation meridian

The pericardium/circulation meridian congestions

Swollen, painful armpits (axillary nodes), skin disorders in the elbow crease and along the meridian. Wrist disorders (such as carpal tunnel syndrome), hyperhidrosis (hot, sweaty palms), arthritis, stiffness or deformities of middle finger, warts, eczema or moles on the middle finger. White spots, fungal growth or ridges on middle finger, as well as whitlows (hang nails).

Internal branch congestions

Diseases of the pericardium and severe disorders of ring finger, such as palmar fibromatosis.

Muscles associated with the pericardium/circulation meridian

GLUTEUS MEDIUS
This is used to pull the leg out sideways and rotate it inwards. If there is weakness in this muscle, the hip and shoulder may be high, and there is also a tendency towards bowed legs or a peculiar limp.[55]

ADDUCTORS
These hold the thigh in and rotate it inward. Weakness can make the pelvis tilt down, will sometimes complicate stiff shoulders and can even cause elbow pain. Problems with the reproductive organs, especially changes in hormone function or menopause, can affect the adductors.[56]

PIRIFORMIS
This hip muscle is very important in posture, especially the position of the sacrum. It is the uppermost of the hip rotators. In a seated position, it allows the leg to move outward. Weakness on one side can cause the

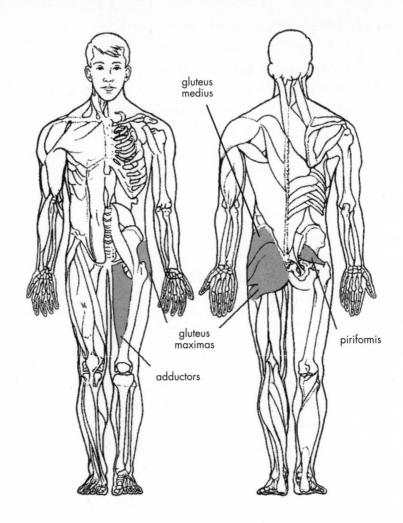

Fig. 24 Muscles associated with the pericardium/circulation

sacrum to twist, making the ankle on that side turn in, the knees 'knock' and the opposite foot turn out. It is located adjacent to the sciatic nerve (the longest, largest nerve in the body), and problems with this muscle can often affect the sciatic nerve. There may be pain down the leg, numbness and tingling of the legs, burning urine and other bladder problems.[57]

GLUTEUS MAXIMUS

This is one of the largest and strongest muscles in the body. It acts as a stabilizer of the lower back and extends the thigh. Weakness of one side will twist the pelvis or make the crease of the buttocks go off to one side. With both sides weak, walking becomes difficult.[58]

The Triple Burner Meridian

The triple burner meridian has an ascending (yang) flow of energy running from the hand to the head. It receives its Chi from the pericardium meridian and passes it on to the gall bladder meridian. The meridian starts on the back of the ring finger, ascends up the arm and ends at the top of the outer corner of the eye (see figure 25).

Says the Nei Ching: 'The three burning spaces are like the officials who plan the construction of ditches and sluices and they create waterways.'[59] The triple burner is not exactly an organ, but a relationship between a number of organs. The Chinese saw it as being composed of three sections which control the chemical activity within the body, regulate and adjust body temperature changes, and transfer Chi from one area to another. The three 'heaters', 'warmers' or 'burners' correspond to three divisions of the body: the upper burner to the thoracic cavity including the heart and lungs; the middle burner to the upper abdominal cavity including the spleen/pancreas and the stomach; and the lower burner to the lower abdominal cavity which encompasses the liver and kidneys, intestines and bladder.[60]

This meridian governs activities involving all the organs and it unites the respiratory, digestive and excretory systems. It may be related to the hypothalamus, the link between the nervous system and endocrine glands. Its functions include:

1   Regulation of the autonomic nervous system, thus of the heart and abdominal organs, especially in their response to emotion.
2   Control of the pituitary (which regulates the output of all the endocrine glands).
3   Regulation of body temperature, appetite and thirst.
4   Control of the emotions and moods, so influencing social relations.[61]

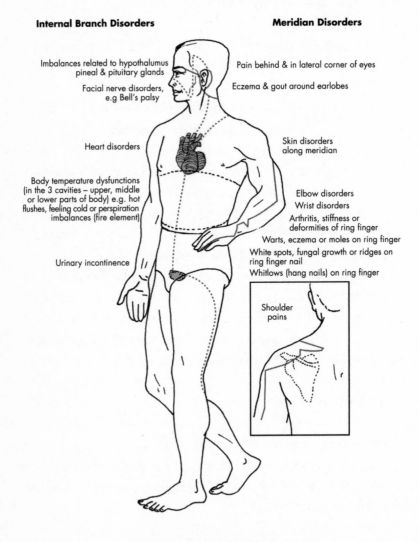

Internal Branch Disorders

Imbalances related to hypothalumus pineal & pituitary glands

Facial nerve disorders, e.g Bell's palsy

Heart disorders

Body temperature dysfunctions (in the 3 cavities – upper, middle or lower parts of body) e.g. hot flushes, feeling cold or perspiration imbalances (fire element)

Urinary incontinence

Meridian Disorders

Pain behind & in lateral corner of eyes

Eczema & gout around earlobes

Skin disorders along meridian

Elbow disorders
Wrist disorders
Arthritis, stiffness or deformities of ring finger
Warts, eczema or moles on ring finger
White spots, fungal growth or ridges on ring finger nail
Whitlows (hang nails) on ring finger

Shoulder pains

Fig. 25 Triple burner meridian

The triple burner meridian congestions

Arthritis, stiffness or deformities of the ring fingers, warts, eczema or moles on the ring fingers as well as white spots, fungal growth or ridges on the ring finger nails. Whitlows (hang nails) on ring fingers. Wrist disorders. Elbow disorders and skin disorders along the meridian. Shoulder pains. Pain behind or in lateral corner of eyes, eczema, as well as gout around earlobes.

Internal branch congestions

Imbalances related to hypothalamus, pineal and pituitary glands. Facial nerve disorders, such as Bell's palsy. Heart disorders and body temperature dysfunctions in the three cavities – upper, middle or lower parts of body – such as hot flushes, feeling cold or perspiration imbalances (fire element). Urinary incontinence.

Muscles associated with the triple burner meridian

TERES MINOR
This is the shoulder muscle which rotates the arm and can be involved in wrist and elbow problems. With weakness on one side, the hands will be turned differently when the arms hang down to the side.[62]

SARTORIUS
This thigh muscle helps to flex the thigh and rotate it outwards. It is the longest muscle in the body. Weakness will cause the pelvis to twist and it can also be the cause of knee pain of knock-knees because of the resulting instability of the knee joint. Adrenal problems can affect this muscle.[63]

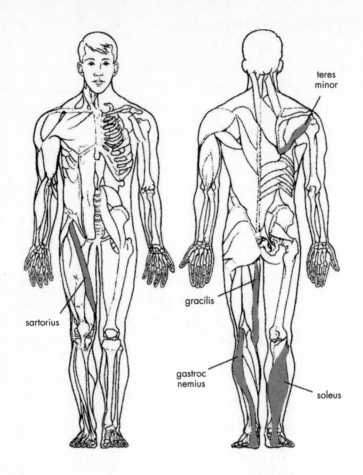

Fig. 26 Muscles associated with the triple burner

GRACILIS

This thigh muscle pulls the leg inwards. When lying down it is the first muscle used when bending the knee. Weakness makes it difficult to bend the knee without flexing the hip. Adrenal problems can be related to this muscle.[64]

SOLEUS

This is the calf muscle which flexes the foot and the lower part of the leg, steadying the foot. Weakness may cause a forward lean of the body or bending of the knees. Adrenal problems can affect this muscle.[65]

GASTROCNEMIUS

This calf muscle works with the soleus in flexing the foot and lower part of the leg. Weakness can cause hyperextension of the knee (knee pushed too far back), inability to rise up on the toes or difficulty bending the knee.[66]

THE WOOD ELEMENT

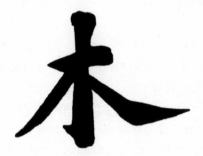

Fig. 27 Wood element

The wood element refers to living, growing entities: trees, plants and the human body. They grow simultaneously out and up, down and in. The development of the root structure, as well as its early nourishment by sun, air, water and soil, provides strength and growth to the organism. Each entity has its individual requirements in these areas. The wood element refers to the growing structures; the roots, trunks and limbs of the trees and plants; the ligaments, tendons and muscles that hold the human body upright and together. A wood imbalance can result in poor flexibility or a 'weak rootedness' in an individual. Arthritis and muscular disorders are viewed as wood problems. The wood element creates our mental clarity and ability to focus, plan and make decisions. A strongly overdeveloped wood element may result in excessive mental activity – for example someone who tries to organize everything and everyone; this person may have a hard time relaxing and be prone to migraines and temple headaches.

The Gall Bladder Meridian

The gall bladder meridian has a descending (yang) flow of energy running from the head to the foot. It receives its Chi from the triple burner meridian and passes it on to the liver meridian. The gall bladder meridian starts at the outer corner of the eye, traverses the temple and descends to the shoulder. It continues laterally down the body and leg to end on the back of the fourth toe, towards the little toe (see figure 28).

'The gall bladder occupies the position of an important and upright official who excels through his decision and judgement,' states the Nei Ching.[67] According to the ancients, the attitudes of all the other organs originate in the energy of the gall bladder. The gall bladder is different from the other organs in that they transport 'impure' or foreign matter – food, liquid and the waste products thereof. Only the gall bladder exclusively transports 'pure' liquids.[68]

The gall bladder stores and secretes bile – a bitter yellow fluid continuously produced by the liver – and sends this bile down into the intestine where it aids the digestive process. Any disruption of the liver will affect the gall bladder's bile secretion and disharmonies of the gall bladder will consequently affect the liver.

This meridian traverses almost the entire body except the arms. It zigzags across the head in a pattern which, in times of stress and tension, becomes like a vice and it is therefore significant in cases of headaches, neck tension and being 'uptight'.[69]

The Nei Ching states that the gall bladder rules decisions, so angry behaviour and rash decisions may indicate an excess of gall bladder Chi, while indecision and timidity may be signs of gall bladder disharmony and weakness.[70]

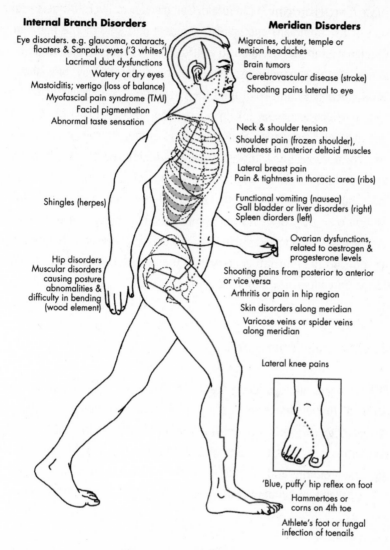

Internal Branch Disorders

Eye disorders. e.g. glaucoma, cataracts, floaters & Sanpaku eyes ('3 whites')
Lacrimal duct dysfunctions
Watery or dry eyes
Mastoiditis; vertigo (loss of balance)
Myofascial pain syndrome (TMJ)
Facial pigmentation
Abnormal taste sensation

Shingles (herpes)

Hip disorders
Muscular disorders causing posture abnomalities & difficulty in bending (wood element)

Meridian Disorders

Migraines, cluster, temple or tension headaches

Brain tumors
Cerebrovascular disease (stroke)
Shooting pains lateral to eye

Neck & shoulder tension
Shoulder pain (frozen shoulder), weakness in anterior deltoid muscles

Lateral breast pain
Pain & tightness in thoracic area (ribs)

Functional vomiting (nausea)
Gall bladder or liver disorders (right)
Spleen diorders (left)

Ovarian dysfunctions, related to oestrogen & progesterone levels

Shooting pains from posterior to anterior or vice versa

Arthritis or pain in hip region

Skin disorders along meridian

Varicose veins or spider veins along meridian

Lateral knee pains

'Blue, puffy' hip reflex on foot
Hammertoes or corns on 4th toe
Athlete's foot or fungal infection of toenails

Fig. 28 Gall bladder meridian

Gall bladder meridian congestions

Shooting pains lateral to the eye; migraines, cluster, temple or tension headaches. Brain tumours and cerebrovascular disease (stroke), neck and shoulder tension (such as frozen shoulder), weakness in anterior deltoid muscles. Lateral breast pain and tightness and pain in the thoracic area (ribs), functional vomiting (nausea). Gall bladder or liver disorders (right side of the meridian) and spleen disorders (left side of the meridian). Ovarian dysfunctions related to oestrogen and progesterone levels. Evidence of these conditions will often be supported by face-shaped brown blemishes on and around the cheekbone – especially if the subject is a female and is taking an oral contraceptive pill or is going through the menopause. Shooting pains from posterior to anterior or vice versa, as well as arthritis or pain in the hip region. Skin disorders, varicose veins or spider veins along the meridian; lateral knee pains. A 'blue, puffy' hip reflex close to the lateral anklebone may be a confirmation of lower back into hip complaints, however, it must be noted that the gall bladder meridian is the underlying concern. Hammertoes or corns on the fourth toes, as well as the potential for athlete's foot or fungal infection of the toenails.

Internal branch congestions

Eye disorders, such as glaucoma, cataracts, floaters and Sanpaku eyes, lacrimal duct dysfunctions, watery or dry eyes; mastoiditis, vertigo (loss of balance), myofascial pain syndrome (TMJ), facial pigmentation and abnormal taste sensation. Shingles on the lateral side of the body (herpes), hip disorders and muscular disorders causing posture abnormalities and difficulty in bending (wood element).

Muscles associated with the gall bladder meridian

ANTERIOR DELTOID
This muscle is used together with the coracobrachialis in flexing the shoulder with the elbow bent, as when combing the hair. It is not usually found to be weak, but could be related to many headache cases, which are caused by toxicity from bad diet.[71]

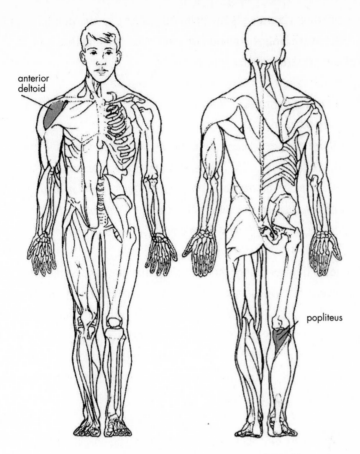

Fig. 29 Muscles associated with the gall bladder

POPLITEUS

This muscle turns the lower leg in. Problems here could be hyperexten-sion of the knee (knee pushed too far back), and bending the knee may become difficult or painful.[72]

The Liver Meridian

The liver meridian has an ascending (yin) flow of energy running from the foot to the chest. It receives Chi from the gall bladder meridian and passes it on to the lung meridian. The liver meridian starts on the back of the big toe and ascends medially up the leg to the genital region. From there it continues upwards to just below the nipple on the lower part of the breastbone. (see figure 30).

The Nei Ching states:

> 'The liver has the functions of a military leader who excels in his strategic planning ... The liver causes utmost weariness and is the dwelling place of the soul, or the spiritual part of man that ascends to heaven. The liver influences the nails and is effective upon the muscles; it brings forth animal desires and vigour.'[73]

According to the Nei Ching, the liver rules 'flowing' and 'spreading'. The liver or liver Chi is responsible for smooth movement of bodily substances and for regularity of body activities. It sends Chi and blood to every part of the body, and maintains evenness and harmony of movement throughout the body. All activity that depends on Chi also depends on the liver. Any impairment of liver function can influence the circulation of Chi and blood.[74]

The liver controls bile secretions and is involved in the storage and regulation of blood. It is the primary centre of metabolism, synthesizing proteins, neutralizing poisons and regulating blood sugar levels; it also stores glycogen (starch), changing it back to glucose (sugar) when needed for energy. Since the brain does not store glucose, a steady supply from the liver is crucial to life, and this is why the ancient Chinese saw the liver as vital to conscious and unconscious thought, and responsible for creating a relaxed internal environment.[75]

Emotional disruptions will affect the functioning of the liver, and this in turn will affect the emotional state. Anger, depression and emotional frustrations are associated with the liver. Balance in this meridian will produce a sense of well-being and equitable temperament.[76] In

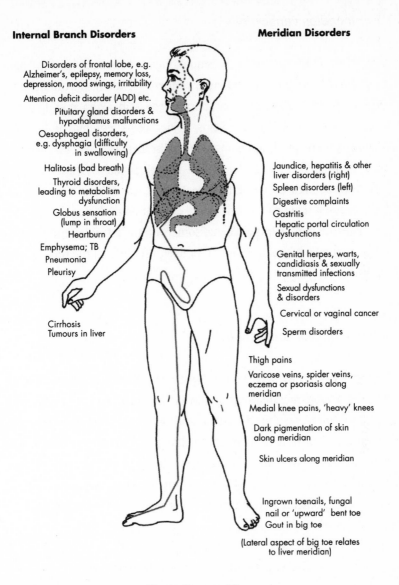

Internal Branch Disorders

Disorders of frontal lobe, e.g. Alzheimer's, epilepsy, memory loss, depression, mood swings, irritability

Attention deficit disorder (ADD) etc.

Pituitary gland disorders & hypothalamus malfunctions

Oesophageal disorders, e.g. dysphagia (difficulty in swallowing)

Halitosis (bad breath)

Thyroid disorders, leading to metabolism dysfunction

Globus sensation (lump in throat)

Heartburn

Emphysema; TB

Pneumonia

Pleurisy

Cirrhosis
Tumours in liver

Meridian Disorders

Jaundice, hepatitis & other liver disorders (right)

Spleen disorders (left)

Digestive complaints

Gastritis

Hepatic portal circulation dysfunctions

Genital herpes, warts, candidiasis & sexually transmitted infections

Sexual dysfunctions & disorders

Cervical or vaginal cancer

Sperm disorders

Thigh pains

Varicose veins, spider veins, eczema or psoriasis along meridian

Medial knee pains, 'heavy' knees

Dark pigmentation of skin along meridian

Skin ulcers along meridian

Ingrown toenails, fungal nail or 'upward' bent toe

Gout in big toe

(Lateral aspect of big toe relates to liver meridian)

Fig. 30 Liver meridian

China, it is said that the liver governs the eyes, and many eye complaints can be related to the liver. The tendons are also related to the liver.

Liver meridian congestions

Symptoms on the big toe such as gout, ingrown toenails, 'upward' bent toe, rigid toe, fungal nails and ingrown toenails; skin ulcers on the inner side of the calf; dark pigmentation of the skin along meridian and medial knee pains. Varicose veins, spider veins, eczema or psoriasis along the meridian. Thigh pains. Sperm disorders (see section on infertility, page 105), cervical or vaginal cancer, sexual dysfunctions and disorders, as well as genital herpes, warts, candidiasis and sexually transmitted infections. Hepatic portal circulation dysfunctions, gastritis and digestive complaints. Spleen disorders on the left side of the meridian and jaundice; hepatitis and other liver disorders on the right side of the meridian.

Internal branch congestions

Disorders of frontal lobe, such as Alzheimer's disease, epilepsy, memory loss, depression, mood swings and irritability; attention deficit disorder (ADD). Pituitary gland disorders and hypothalamus malfunctions. Oesophageal disorders, such as dysphagia (difficulty in swallowing); halitosis (bad breath), thyroid disorders leading to metabolism dysfunction and globus sensation (lump in throat). Heartburn, emphysema, tuberculosis, pneumonia and pleurisy. Cirrhosis and liver tumours.

Did you know? – Depression and diet

Research has found that depression is more widespread than coronary heart disease, cancer and AIDS – and is just as costly to the society. Absenteeism and lost productivity account for more than half these costs. Depression is twice as common in women as in men, and seems to be particularly prevalent after childbirth and during menopause. However, depressed men are twice as likely to suffer from impotence with loss of libido, difficulty in achieving an erection, frigidity and premature ejaculation all telltale signs. A survey reported that nearly half of all men and a quarter of all women who are on anti-depression medication report problems in their sex lives. The survey showed that 45% of men and 27% of women experience sexual problems once they begin taking anti-depression drugs.

Nowadays, children are prescribed Prozac for any number of personality and behaviour problems, including depression, separation anxiety, shyness, obsessive-compulsive behaviour and eating disorders. Others are given the stimulant Ritalin for hyperactivity and conduct disorders. While 30 years ago, it was not recognized that children can become depressed, it is now widely accepted.

Many believe that the answers to emotional health are to be found in the combination of body chemistry and environment. The following are characteristic warning signals:

- Feelings of worthlessness, guilt and self-blame, as well as feeling out of control and unable to cope;
- Tiredness, loss of energy and a general feeling of lethargy;
- Suicidal thoughts;
- Poor concentration, forgetfulness, indecisiveness and difficulty expressing oneself;
- Loss of appetite and weight or, conversely, an increase in appetite and weight gain;
- Changes in sleep patterns – insomnia or hypersomnia (sleeping more than usual);

- Unusual agitation and restlessness or, conversely, a slow-ing down of all reactions.

Keeping in mind that the liver and gall bladder represent the wood element, it is clear that the quality of food intake in any form – even the chemical intake of drugs – is particularly relevant here. The nutrition guru and author Patrick Holford says that eating the right food is scientifically proven to boost your IQ, improve your mood, increase your energy levels, boost your memory and keep your mind ever young. In his book Optimum Nutrition for the Mind, he lists five essential 'brain foods':

- Complex carbohydrates – such as whole grains, beans, nuts and seeds; fruits and vegetables are another good source as they are good foundations of the most important nutrient of all for the brain and nervous system: glucose, the fuel (wood) they run on.
- Smart fats – are the essential fatty acids, omega-3 and omega-6, that are the 'architects of higher intelligence'. They have to be topped up through diet. Other than the water, our brains are 60% fat.
- Phospholipids – are the 'intelligent' fats in your brain, the memory's 'best friends'. The richest sources are egg yolks and offal.
- Amino acids – are the 'alphabet of mind and mood', the building blocks of protein that improve the brain's talking. The words the brain uses to send messages from one cell to another are neurotransmitters and the letters they are built from are amino acids – obtained from vegetables and animals sources.

- Intelligent nutrients – are vitamins and minerals that are the brain's 'master tuners' and 'best friends'. These include B vitamins, manganese and zinc. The brain needs vitamins and minerals to turn glucose into energy.

Muscles associated with the liver meridian

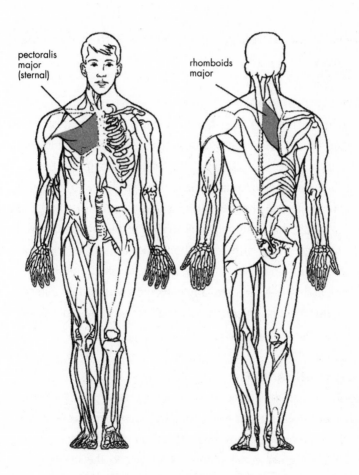

pectoralis major (sternal)

rhomboids major

Fig. 31 Muscles associated with the liver

PECTORALIS MAJOR (STERNAL)

This is responsible for moving the arm in, turning and drawing it forward.[77]

RHOMBOIDS

These muscles, in the back of the shoulders, pull the shoulder blades together and upwards. They are used with the levator scapulae and are rarely found to be weak.[78]

The behavioural patterns of the individual with wood element imbalances

THE SEASON: SPRING

The beginning of spring is 21 March in the Northern hemisphere and 21 September in the Southern hemisphere, the time of spring equinox when the length of day equals night. Just as spring is a time when nature is 'budding' and coming alive – we are likely to experience a new spark of life and are filled with inspiration and new energy to act upon our ideas. This is a good time to look at our life and make new plans. However, those with congestions and lack of Chi feel ill and a sense that everything inside of them is dead, finished. The spring within them is asking to be created. Some people say that their ailments or depressions are worse in spring – or that spring is the only time they feel good.

THE EMOTION: ANGER

A person with an imbalance in the wood element will have a marked presence of anger in themselves; they will often be on edge with others and pick a fight for no apparent reason. An imbalance results in aggression, difficulty in calming one's anger and the tendency to hit out in rage at anything in one's reach. Everyone gets angry at times, but if this condition is continuous it is likely to indicate an imbalance in the wood element. Balance in this element produces patience and good spirits. A strong wood element is evident in a flexible approach when confronted by the pressures of life. This type of person is able to make complex life decisions, plan ahead and execute their plans efficiently, rather than being emotionally stuck or 'green with envy' (see 'Colour' below). Increasingly, there appears to be widespread anger and dissatisfaction amongst individuals and wider populations. (See section on Sanpaku eyes for more on anger outbursts, pages 166–8.)

THE TIME OF DAY OF PEAK: GALL BLADDER 11PM–1AM; LIVER 1–3AM

People with a wood element imbalance and congestions along the two related meridians often suffer from insomnia – and if they cannot sleep in the early hours of the morning, the insomnia is a confirmation of an imbalance in the wood element. The gall bladder meridian passes over the lateral sides of the head/brain and it is interesting to note that the Chinese relate the gall bladder to the ability of making decisions. Many individuals when confronted with major decisions will often use the expression 'I'll sleep on it': if their wood element is unbalanced they are more likely to experience insomnia and a night of tossing and turning, feeling no clearer about the correct decision in the morning; however, someone with balanced energy in the wood element will have a peaceful sleep and almost dream of the decisions and wake with the knowledge of their direction.

THE SOUND: SHOUTING

A subtle pervasive tone in a person's voice; whatever a person says is a kind of shout, aggressive and forceful. On entering a room, you can often quickly identify those with wood element by hearing a piercing voice amongst the group. However, a person who speaks with timid manner or has to repeat the sentences may have a weakness in the wood element. Nonetheless, it is important to remember this is a clear cry for help.

THE TISSUES: LIGAMENTS, TENDONS AND MUSCLES

A forward bending person, a person with muscular diseases or someone with weak physical strength are confirming an imbalance with the wood element. Our feet represent the root system of a strong tree and in nature a tree sometimes has to be supported against the environment with ropes until it is strong and well rooted; the same principle should apply to a 'weak' human being. Good quality supporting shoes, perhaps with insoles, might be the best solution until the wood element has become stronger through lifestyle changes.

Did you know? – People as trees

A person can be compared to a tree; capable of withstanding life's seasonal changes, strong yet flexible without becoming uprooted. Being the strong tree makes us able to make decisions and plan ahead; establishing roots that will supply us with nourishment and continue the cycle of procreation and prevent us getting swayed by the wind of change or 'break' us, enabling us to adapt to our circumstances without being rigid, angry and on edge with loved ones and society as a whole.

If a tree/person is planted in the incorrect environment and is not receiving the correct nourishment and sunlight (love) required for growth and strength, it will lose its vitality. The roots will not grow deep enough to withstand the storms and support the trunk. The tree will not be structured, strong or symmetrical and will be unable to grow, procreate and survive. The branches of the tree will become weak, the person feel stiff in the muscles, ligaments and tendons and the posture changes. Without flexibility, easily uprooted and pushed over when faced with the pressures in life, a person is unable to adapt to the changes in life and this makes for indecisiveness.

These weaknesses are often reflected in the feet. The feet mirror the body and a person with an imbalanced wood element is frequently rigid with high arches or, alternatively, the feet are very flat and inflexible. The ligaments and tendons in the toes are usually shortened, causing the toes to be clawed, making for a weak 'root' system.

THE EXTERNAL PHYSICAL MANIFESTATION: THE NAILS

The colouring, white spots, fungal growth, indentations and vertical ridges of the nails can give evidence as to the body's nourishment – and therefore of the quality of our wood intake. For example, vertical ridges on the fingernails give an indication of high acid-forming foods; however, each of the elements manifest in some way on the nails so it is important to take note on which fingernail/s the ridges are on. White spots appear on the nails when there is a high intake of sugary foods or stimulants which deplete the mineral content of our cells. Indentations in the nails happen when severe changes in lifestyle have occurred or when we are ill and have been given strong medication. Ingrown toenails, especially on the big toe – the spleen/pancreas meridian on the outer side, and the liver meridian on the inner side towards the second – give evidence of low Chi in the related meridian. Ingrown toenails can also appear on other toes, such as the second toe representing the stomach meridian or the fourth toe being the gall bladder meridian.

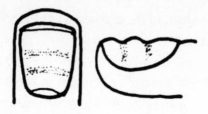

Fig. 32a Nail with indentations

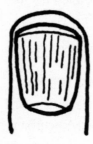

Fig. 32b Nail with vertical ridges

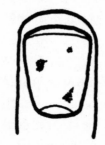

Fig. 32c Nail with white spots

THE SENSE ORGAN: THE EYES

The sense of sight relates to the balance of Chi within the wood element. All the eye disorders that impair the sight are therefore evidence of wood imbalance, such as short and long sightedness, cataracts, glaucoma, floaters and blindness, as well as the phenomena of 'Sanpaku' eyes (see below).

Did you know? – Sanpaku eyes

Abnormal expansion and contraction of the eyeballs produces a condition known as 'Sanpaku', a Japanese word meaning 'three whites'. In a normal eye, the upper and lower eyelids should cover the top and bottom of the irises. The only areas of white that should be visible are on either side

of the iris. If it is possible to see the white of the eyes in three
areas – both sides and top, or both sides and bottom – then
that person has developed 'Sanpaku' eyes.

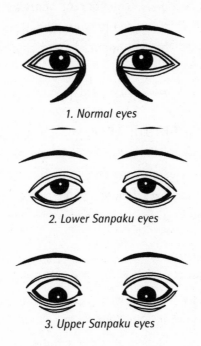

1. Normal eyes

2. Lower Sanpaku eyes

3. Upper Sanpaku eyes

Fig. 33 Sanpaku eyes

Contracted eyeballs, which are normal in infants and young
children, produce upper 'Sanpaku' (upper whites showing). If
this condition continues beyond early childhood, or begins
at a later stage, it is a sign of a seriously imbalanced nervous
system. Such a person's mind, body and spirit are out of harmony and the intuitive skills are usually out of touch. This
condition also shows that the nerve cells are expanding,
often resulting in abnormal behaviour and thinking (such as
aggression, violence and uncontrollable passions). Lower
'Sanpaku' (the lower whites showing) is caused by the
abnormal expansion of the eyeballs. Again, the nerve cells of

the brain are expanded, resulting in abnormal behaviour and thinking and may lead to great vulnerability.

Note: When facing this condition of upper or lower 'San-paku' eyes, there is no need to worry unduly. The condition can be reversed through improving and changing current lifestyle habits.

THE FLUID SECRETION: THE TEARS

People who are suffering from dry eyes and constantly use eye drops, blaming such factors as air conditioning or the dry climate, or, conversely, people whose eyes frequently feel watery, especially when walking in the wind (see below), confirm a wood imbalance.

THE FLAVOUR: SOUR

When we serve lemon with fatty seafoods, the sour ingredient helps the liver digest fatty foods. However, people who crave sour-tasting foods or look to add sour ingredients to their food are demonstrating that they have liver problems and are attempting to remedy the situation by using plenty of sour ingredients as 'medicine'. In the early stage of pregnancy, some women crave sour ingredients and, for instance, will eat a jar of gherkins or eat lemons as if they were oranges, again confirming stress with the function of the liver meridian. A total dislike and inability to eat even slightly sour foods also signifies an imbalance.

THE SMELL: RANCID

The Nei Ching also describes this smell as offensive and fetid; elsewhere it is described as urine or sour sweet. These smells are difficult to define and each individual's perception of them will be slightly different.

THE CLIMATE: THE WIND

One sometimes hears expressions such as 'I can feel it in my big toe – the weather is going to change' or 'The wind brings on my migraine'. (It is interesting to note here that the big toe relates to both the liver and spleen/pancreas meridians.) Keeping in mind that the meridians are electromagnetic in character, the wind is also electrically charged (particularly the winds associated with thunder and lightning storms), and if there are congestions along the meridians, the symptoms will be exacerbated during changes in the weather. The congestion 'gout' that is mostly manifested in the big toe often hurts during such storms.

THE COLOUR: GREEN

'Green with envy' is an expression often used, however the ancient Chinese related the colour to imbalances with the wood element and envy as a form of anger – also relating to the wood element. Still, a green hue in the face points to the wood element, as does preference of the use of the green colour in clothing and interior designs to the exclusion of other colours; conversely, if the green colour is detested to the extreme this also points to a wood imbalance.

THE SPECIAL MERIDIANS

Two special meridians, referred to as 'vessels' – the governing vessel and conception vessel – are considered major meridians. This is because they have independent points – points that are not on any of the 12 other meridians.[78] These two vessels run along the midline of the body – front and back – to form what seems to be the central body circuit. They are not part of the general meridian circulatory system but are related to it as a secondary channel.[80]

Governing Vessel

A yang meridian, this acts mainly on the yang energy, having a governing effect on all the other yang meridians and organs – small intestine,
triple burner, stomach, large intestine, bladder and gall bladder. The
yang organ functions are primarily active and relate to the breaking
down of food and fluids and the absorption of nutrients from them, the
circulation of the derived 'nourishing energies' around the body, and
the secretion of unused materials.[81] The three yang meridians found in
the feet are the largest, covering a large portion of the body. When the
body is bent forward, the meridians have an 'outside' path, which is
characteristic of yang meridians. The energy flow is ascendant, running
from the coccyx to the upper gum.

The governing vessel begins in the pelvic cavity, and ascends along the
middle of the spinal column to penetrate the brain. The main branch
continues over the top of the head, descends across the forehead and
nose to end inside the upper gum. An internal branch starts in the
pelvic cavity and ascends through the tip of the coccyx to reach the
kidneys in the lumbar region (see figure 35).[82]

Right on the top of the head is a special connecting point for all yang
meridians. According to Chinese philosophy, it is a point of contact of
the heavenly yang. The name of the point is 'Baihui' which means
'meeting point for 100 points'. This point governs all other points and
meridians in the body.[83]

Muscle associated with the governing vessel

TERES MAJOR
This muscle in the back of the shoulder draws the arm in and keeps it
turned out.[84]

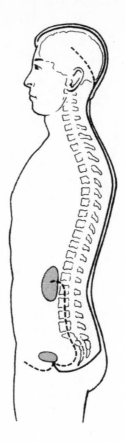

Fig. 34 Governing vessel

CONCEPTION VESSEL

This is a yin vessel, which has a governing effect on all the other yin meridians. Via its connection with the yin meridians from the foot, it has a special effect on the lowest of the three burners, and thereby on the ability to conceive. The yin meridians and organ functions – heart, pericardium, spleen/pancreas, lungs, kidneys and liver – are related to the storing of vital essence. They have to do with the generation, regulation, transformation and storage of energy, blood, fluids, and spirit (shen). Yin functions are conceived of as deeper and more essential for vital functioning than the yang functions.[85] The energy flow is ascendant, running from the perineum to the chin.

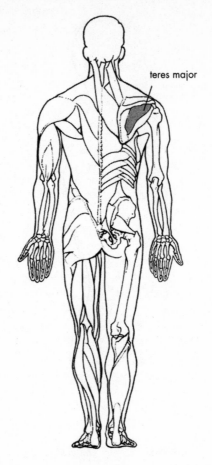

teres major

Fig. 35 Muscles associated with the governing vessel

The conception vessel starts from the pelvic cavity and runs forward across the pubic region. It ascends along the midline of the abdomen, through the chest. It then passes up the throat to the lower jaw. An internal branch encircles the lips and branches lip to the eyes[86] (see figure 36). The special connecting point for all yin meridians is situated at the base of the sternum where, according to the Nei Ching, all the energies are collected.

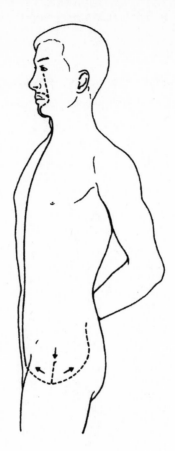

Fig. 36 Conception vessel

Muscle associated with the conception vessel

SUPRASPINATUS

This muscle helps in moving the arm away from the body and in holding the arm into the shoulder socket, so it can be involved in shoulder problems.[87]

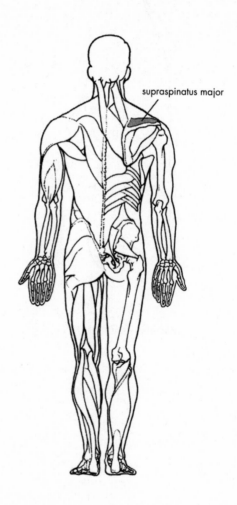

supraspinatus major

Fig. 37 Muscles associated with the conception vessel

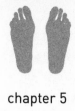

chapter 5

mapping the feet

The head and feet keep warm
The rest will take no harm

ANON

Mapping the Reflexes on the Feet

Understanding the structure of the feet in relation to the body is the first and most important step to understanding reflexology. It is, in fact, very simple, as the feet are a microcosm or mini-map of the whole body and all the organs and body parts are reflected on the feet in a similar arrangement as in the body. These reflexes are found on the plantar and dorsal aspects and along the medial and lateral sides of the feet, and their positions follow a logical anatomical pattern.

The body itself is divided horizontally into four parts:

1   The head and neck area;
2   The thoracic area from the shoulders to the diaphragm;
3   The abdominal area from the diaphragm to the pelvic area;
4   The pelvis.

These areas can be delineated clearly on the feet and provide a precise picture of the body as it is reflected on the feet. In view of this it is simplest to examine the situation of body organs in horizontal divisions. This is easier to understand if looked at together with the meridians.

The sections described above are also clearly visible in the foot structure:

- The head and neck area = the toes;
- The thoracic area = the ball of the foot;
- The abdominal area = the arch;
- The pelvic area = the heel;
- The reproductive area = the ankle;
- The spine = the medial foot;
- The outer body = the lateral foot;
- Circulation and breasts = dorsal aspect of the feet.

Mapping the Reflexes on the Feet According to a Mirror Image of the Meridians

Seeing that in this book we have progressed away from the historical link to the zones, it is also useful to map the reflexes on the feet as a reflection of the meridians. In my first book on reflexology, I established the concept that the sections of the meridians found in the torso, and therefore the related organs, are what should be reflected on the foot and the reflexes. Careful study of the meridian pathways and related organs will clarify organ location on reflexology charts and explain how organ reflexes relate to the meridians. Meridians do not run in straight lines – zones do.

To establish how reflexes, meridians and organs are connected, we should look first at the toes. The second and third toes correspond to the eye reflexes, the fourth and fifth toes to the ear reflexes. The tips of

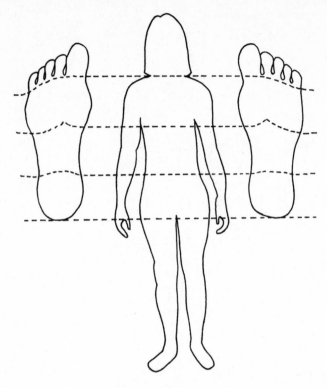

Fig. 1 Division of the body

all the toes represent the sinus reflexes. When relating meridians to the situation of the reflexes, parallels can be drawn.

The most relevant meridian is the stomach meridian. This has its origin under the eyes, lateral to the nose. It has a descending pathway, which ends in the second toe – the eye reflex. One of the internal branches ends in the third toe – also the eye reflex. The curved path of the stomach meridian affects the sinuses, throat, lungs, diaphragm, spleen (left side), liver, gall bladder (right side), stomach, pancreas, duodenum, adrenal glands, kidneys, large intestine, small intestine and pelvic region. All the reflexes of these organs are situated beneath the second and third toes – the stomach meridians, except the spleen reflex, which is situated mainly below the fourth toe. The zig-zag pathway of the meridian is evident on the torso as well as the feet.

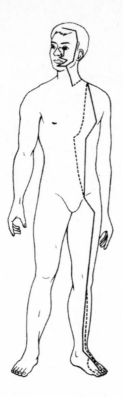

Fig. 2 Stomach meridian

The gall bladder meridian begins in the face next to the eyes and descends on the lateral aspect of the body to end in the fourth toe. It circulates around the ear, and therefore directly relates to the ear reflex, which is situated on the fourth toe – however, sense of hearing belongs to the water element. The internal branch meridian is represented in the big toe (towards the second toe), which relates to the mastoid and Eustachian tube reflexes – linking the first toe to the fourth toe. The gall bladder meridian penetrates lateral portions of the lungs, liver, gall bladder (right side), spleen (left side), large intestine and lateral hip area. According to reflexology charts, the reflexes for a part of all these organs are situated below the fourth toe, and to the lateral side of the foot. The liver and spleen/pancreas meridians both begin in the big toe and end in the breast region. Both meridians have internal branches, which run

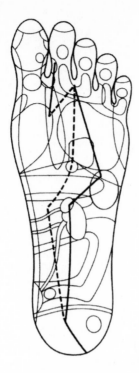

Fig. 3 Part of the stomach meridian mirrored onto the foot

through the throat area, and therefore indirectly affect the throat and thyroid (see figures 3a,b below). The thyroid is also affected by the stomach meridian, as mentioned above. Bunions are usually situated on the spleen/pancreas meridian and around the thyroid reflex, and therefore also concern the thyroid. Some authors of reflexology find the thyroid is 'helped' when reflexes on the second toe and around the big toe are worked on. These reflexes are often sensitive if there are thyroid disorders. This is again due to stimulation of the meridians.

The thyroid reflex has been repositioned by some authors, at the area near the big toe – the neck area (see figure 4). This is probably because in this position it fits in more accurately with the image of the body stipulated in zone therapy. However, most charts and books have retained this as a thyroid 'helper' area as it was realized that working on

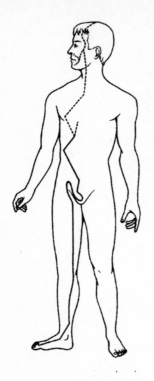

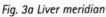

Fig. 3a Liver meridian

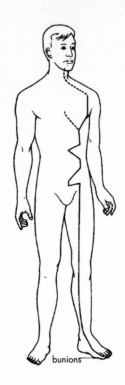

Fig. 3b Spleen/pancreas meridian

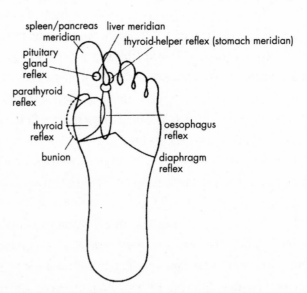

Fig. 3c Positions of reflexes and meridians on the foot

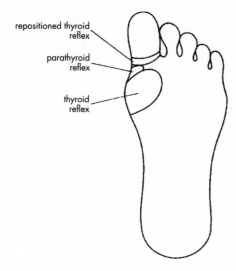

repositioned thyroid reflex

parathyroid reflex

thyroid reflex

Fig. 4 Position of the thyroid reflex

the old reflex area (on the ball of the foot, directly below the big toe) was effective in alleviating thyroid complaints.

According to all reflexology charts, the big toe incorporates the head and brain reflexes. Two important glands – namely the pituitary and pineal glands – are situated in the brain, so their reflexes are found in the brain reflex area of the big toe. Relating this to meridians – the pituitary gland is situated on the liver meridian, the internal branch of which runs through the throat, as well as the frontal lobe and brain (see figures 3a–c above).

Note the position of the uterus/prostate reflexes between the heel and anklebone on the medial side of the foot. The main reason why this area is effective in complaints relating to the uterus and prostate is the presence of the kidney meridian. The kidney meridian also penetrates the uterus/prostate in the body, and according to Chinese medicine the kidneys store the jing – a vital essence involved in reproduction.

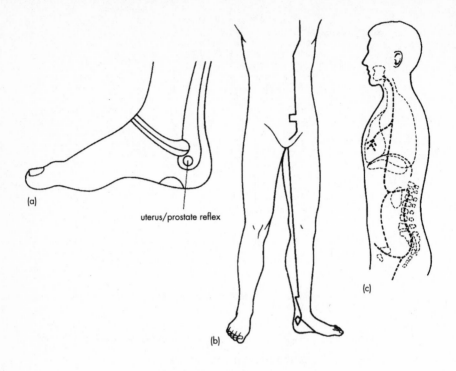

(a)

uterus/prostate reflex

(b)

(c)

Fig. 5a Position of the uterus/prostate reflex

Fig. 5b Section of the kidney meridian

Fig. 5c Internal branch of the kidney meridian

The kidney meridian also exerts an indirect effect on these organs via the internal branch meridian, which runs through the lumbar vertebrae. The nerves from the lumbar vertebrae also serve these organs. It is therefore understandable why many women suffer back problems during menstruation and when giving birth.

The reflexes for the ovaries/testes are situated between the heel and anklebone on the lateral side of the foot. The bladder meridian runs through this area of the foot influencing these reflexes; it also runs through the lumbar vertebrae, and, as with the kidneys, the nerves also serve these organs. On many charts, reflexes for chronic sciatica, uterus, prostate and rectum (anus) are situated on both sides of the Achilles

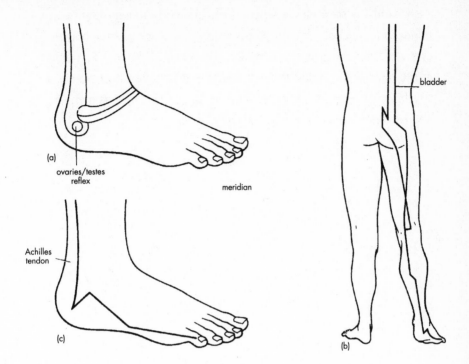

Fig. 6a Position of the ovaries/testes reflex

Fig. 6b Section of the bladder meridian

Fig. 6c Section of the bladder meridian on the foot

tendon. As this area incorporates the kidney and bladder meridians, stimulation here has an effect on everything along these meridian paths.

The heart reflex has been repositioned on many new charts to the area where I have placed the thyroid reflex – again, probably to fit in with zone therapy mapping. Prior to its repositioning, the heart reflex was placed where I describe it. Apart from the uterus/prostate, small intestine and other organs, the kidney meridian also passes through the solar plexus and the lungs. A small internal meridian passes through the heart, and another internal section through the parathyroid. When mirrored on to the feet, this part of the meridian, plus one of its small branches, overlap at the kidney meridian. The kidney meridian starts in the foot at the solar plexus reflex. The heart reflex, though slightly up to one side, touches the solar plexus reflex. One of the internal branches starts from the little toe, runs across the ball of the foot and ends at the solar plexus reflex. It penetrates the heart reflex. In the body, a small internal branch also penetrates the heart. The pancreas meridian also has an internal section penetrating the heart.

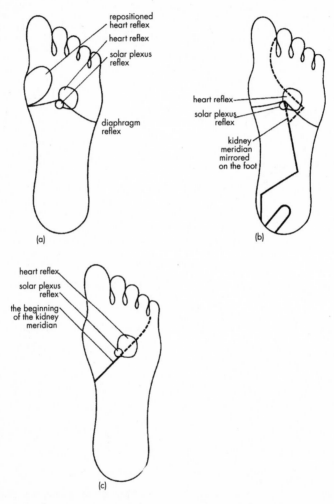

Fig. 7a Position of the heart reflex

Fig. 7b Section of the kidney meridian mirrored on the foot

Fig. 7c Beginning of the kidney meridian

To take this concept of mapping the feet further, take note of the sciatic nerve, which is mapped as a reflex in a band running horizontally across the heel. This is not only a reflex – part of the actual nerve is situated in the heel. Massage to this area often relieves sciatic problems. This is because the bladder meridian runs along the same pathway as the sciatic nerve, and massage here stimulates both the bladder meridian and the sciatic nerve.

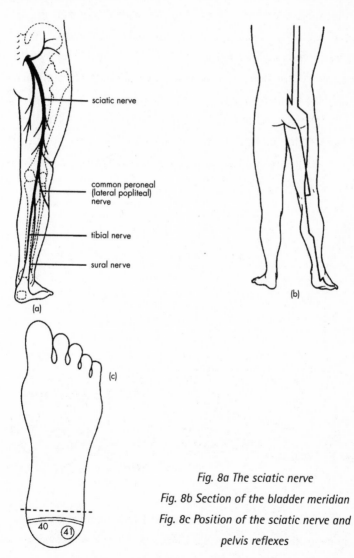

Fig. 8a The sciatic nerve

Fig. 8b Section of the bladder meridian

Fig. 8c Position of the sciatic nerve and

pelvis reflexes

The band across the top of the ankle, from medial to lateral anklebones, represents reflexes for the groin lymph system. All six meridians located in the feet run through the pelvic region, so problems here can be traced to a specific area and meridian.

The bladder meridian, together with the governing vessel, is the only meridian that runs along the spine, and therefore has a profound effect on the spinal cord and nerves. It is the longest meridian in the body, touches all the vertebrae and enters the brain. It therefore concerns the central nervous system and, via the nerve supply, indirectly affects all the organs in the body. The two extra meridians, the 'vessel' meridians, should also be mentioned. The governing vessel runs along the spinal cord at the back of the body, the conception vessel runs midline along the front of the body, thus forming a circuit. This is clearly depicted if the foot is mirrored on to a side view of the body showing these meridians (see figure 9).

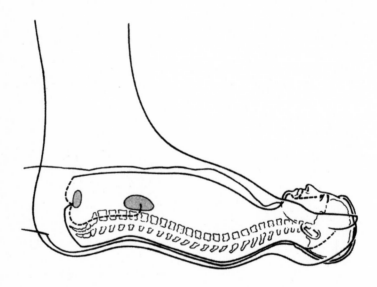

Fig. 9 The foot mirrored on the body showing the governing vessel, which runs along the spinal cord, and the conception vessel, which runs along the front of the foot

The meridians situated in the arms do not penetrate any major organs as they run from face to fingers and vice versa, however their organs and systems are all penetrated by the main six meridians of the feet.

It is thus clear that the reflexes on the feet are closely related to the meridian pathways, and this indicates why a study of meridians should be incorporated with reflexology. This may help explain why it has become more usual to stimulate the reflexes of the feet, rather than their mirror image found on the hands. It may be significant that there are very few books on 'hand reflexology' compared with those on 'foot reflexology'.

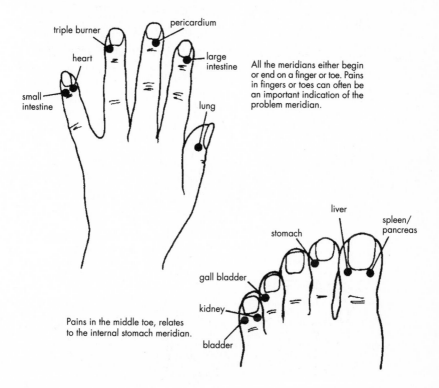

Fig. 10 Correspondence between meridians, toes and fingers

The Head and Neck Area – the Toes

The toes incorporate reflexes to all parts of the body found above the shoulder girdle. If you imagine the two big toes as two half heads with a common neck, the positions of the reflexes are placed logically. Some reflexes overlap, as the organs do in the body. Each big toe contains reflex points for the pituitary gland, pineal gland, hypothalamus, brain, temples, teeth, the seven cervical (neck) vertebrae, sinuses, mastoid, tonsils, nose, mouth and other face reflexes, as well as part of the Eustachian tubes.

The other four toes on each foot contain reflex points for the eyes, ears, teeth, sinuses, lachrymal glands (tear ducts), speech centre, upper lymph system, collarbone (shoulder girdle), Eustachian tubes, chronic eyes and ears.

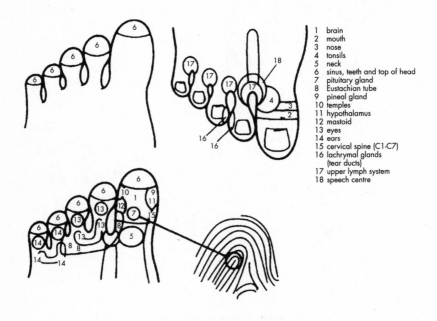

1   brain
2   mouth
3   nose
4   tonsils
5   neck
6   sinus, teeth and top of head
7   pituitary gland
8   Eustachian tube
9   pineal gland
10 temples
11 hypothalamus
12 mastoid
13 eyes
14 ears
15 cervical spine (C1-C7)
16 lachrymal glands
    (tear ducts)
17 upper lymph system
18 speech centre

Fig. 11 The head and neck area

Reflexes of the head and the brain

Reflexes of the head and brain are on the pads of the big toes from the tip behind the nail down over the metatarsal bone; reflexes for the lateral sides of the head and brain are on the sides of the big toes. On the dorsal aspect of the toes, are the face reflexes including the mouth, nose, teeth and tonsils. At the base of the big toe are the neck reflexes.

THE PITUITARY GLAND

This gland, known also as the 'master gland', is considered the most important in the body as it controls the functions of all the endocrine glands. About the size and shape of a cherry, the pituitary gland is attached to the base of the brain. This gland produces numerous hormones – these influence growth, sexual development, metabolism, pregnancy, mineral and sugar content of the blood, fluid retention and energy levels.

The reflex point is found on both feet where the whorl of the big toe print converges into a central point. This is usually situated on the inner side of the toe and often requires a little searching. More often than not, this reflex is found to be off-centre. Since the hormonal system is extremely sensitive and easily thrown off-balance, this reflex is usually very tender.

THE HYPOTHALAMUS

A number of bodily activities are controlled by this part of the brain. It regulates the autonomic nervous system and controls emotional reactions, appetite, body temperature and sleep. The hypothalamus reflex areas are found on both feet on the outer side and tip of the big toe – the same reflex point as the pineal gland.

THE PINEAL GLAND

The pineal gland is a small gland situated within the hypothalamus section of the brain. Its functions are not completely understood but it is known to stimulate the cells in the skin to produce the black pigment melanin. It is thought to play a part in mood and circadian rhythms, and is sometimes referred to as the psychic 'third eye'. The reflexes are on both feet on the outer tip of the big toes – the same as the hypothalamus reflex.

Meridians: The big toe has two meridians, namely the spleen/pancreas on the outer side and the liver meridian on the inner side. The liver meridian corresponds to the wood element that 'feeds' the fire element. It is interesting to note that the fire element represents the triple burner (endocrine) that in the brain comprises of the pituitary gland, pineal and hypothalamus. Many hormonal imbalances, such as problems with the temperature of the body, metabolism, appetite, emotional reactions and sleep, can be directly related to an improper quality of wood (food) on the fire.

The internal branch of the liver meridian penetrates the frontal lobe of the brain and therefore has a direct link to disorders relating to this section, as well as the hormonal glands. The pituitary gland also has an influence on sexual development and it is interesting to note the liver meridian penetrates the sexual organs. The spleen/pancreas meridian relates to the mouth, hence too much or too little salvia relates to an earth element imbalance, as do dry, cracked and swollen lips.

SINUSES

The sinuses are cavities within the skull bones in the brain situated above and to the sides of the nose, in the cheekbones and behind the eyebrows. They communicate with the nasal cavities through small openings. They act as protection for the eyes and the brain and give resonance to the voice. They warm and moisten the air. The reflexes are situated on the tips of all the toes.

Meridians: The sinuses' cavities are penetrated by the stomach meridian – however, forehead sinus congestions are found on the bladder meridian.

TEETH

The reflexes to the teeth are exactly distributed over all the toes: Incisors on the big toe; incisors and canine teeth on the second toe; premolars on the third toe; molars on the fourth toe; wisdom teeth on the fifth toe. These reflexes are in the same position as the sinus reflexes.

Meridians: Teething problems are influenced by the stomach meridians. Many infants are found to be teething and develop nappy rash at the same time. This combination may be assessed as high acid level, congesting the stomach meridian, making the gums sore and the urine more acidic – hence a rash. Grinding of the teeth is related to the same problem. The qualities of the teeth are related to the water element that controls the hard connective tissues such as the teeth, bones and nails. However, the control cycle of the Five Elements indicates that earth controls or loses control of water, meaning high acid levels weaken the hard connective tissues – including the teeth.

EYES

The nerve tissue of the retina receives impressions of images via the pupils and the lens. From there the optic nerve conveys the impressions to the visual area of the cerebral cortex where they are interpreted.

The reflexes are on both feet on the cushions of the second and third toes and may extend slightly down the toes. Reflexes for chronic eye conditions are on the 'shelf' at the base of these two toes.

Meridians: Eye reflexes are found on the second and third toes, where the stomach meridian is also situated. Any problems with the eyes in regards to their appearance, such as conjunctivitis and exophthalmos (protrusion of eyeballs), are due to an imbalance of the acid level in the stomach. However, the sense of seeing or disorders that impair the sense of seeing relate to the wood element and the internal section of the gall bladder meridian that ends under the eyes.

The reflexes for the lachrymal glands (tear ducts) are found on the inside of the second and third toes next to the eye reflexes. However, the wood element looks after the fluid of the eyes and so conditions such as dry or watery eyes are related to an imbalance in this element. In addition, an internal gall bladder meridian section penetrates the eyes at the lachrymal glands.

EARS

The ear is a highly complex system of cavities, bones and membranes, constructed in such a way that sound waves are received and transmitted to the hearing centre in the temporal lobe of the cerebral cortex. The ear also plays a part in maintaining balance.

The reflexes are situated on both feet on the cushions of the fourth and fifth toes and may extend slightly down the toes. The reflexes for the Eustachian tubes extend from the inner side of the big toe along the base of the second and third toes to the fourth toe. Reflexes for chronic ear conditions are found on the 'shelf' at the base of these two toes – the same section as the Eustachian tubes. The mastoid – the part of the skull behind the ear, which contains the air spaces that communicate with the ear – is also treated on these reflexes.

Meridians: Sense of hearing relates to the water element and the fifth toe is where the kidney and bladder meridians end. The bladder meridian has a small internal section going to the ear. Ear problems concerning waxing, inflammation and balance relate to the gall bladder meridian found in the fourth toe; a small internal section goes through the inside of the big toe covering the mastoid reflex. Tinnitus relates to the small intestine meridian – being one of the fire elements – however, wood generates fire, and consequently is an underlying source.

TONSILS

These paired organs are composed of lymphatic tissue and are thought to help protect the throat area. The reflexes are found on both feet – on the top of the foot at the base of the big toe near the web between the big and second toes.

Meridians: Both liver and stomach meridians, in the big and second toes, are involved with problems of the tonsils. Though mostly related to the stomach meridian – the wood (food) controls or loses control of the earth (acid imbalances).

THE LYMPHATIC SYSTEM

The lymphatic system is a network of lymphatic vessels situated throughout the body, which drain tissue fluid surrounding the cells in the body. Lymph nodes filter the lymph to prevent infection passing into the bloodstream and add lymphocytes, which are important for the formation of antibodies and immunological reactions. The main sites of the lymph nodes are in the neck, armpit, breast, abdomen, groin and pelvis, and behind the knees.

On the front of the foot, the webs between the toes are the reflexes for lymph drainage in the neck and chest region of the body. Lymph reflexes for the groin area are linked to the reproductive system and are found in the same area as the reflexes for the Fallopian tubes and vas deferens (see page 206). These reflexes run across the top of the foot from the medial anklebone to the lateral anklebone and incorporate the six main meridians. Congestions in the groin area can be traced to a specific meridian and its organ depending on where exactly these are situated.

The Thoracic Area – the Ball of the Foot

This section of the foot corresponds with the thoracic area in the body from the shoulder girdle to the diaphragm. Several vital reflexes are situated here: the heart, lungs, oesophagus, trachea, bronchi, thyroid and thymus glands, diaphragm and solar plexus.

The thymus gland, oesophagus, trachea and bronchi

The thymus gland is situated in the thoracic cavity. It is quite large in childhood, reaching maximum size at 10–12 years of age, then slowly regresses and almost disappears in adult life. It is involved in the immune system, but its only known function is the formation of lymphocytes.

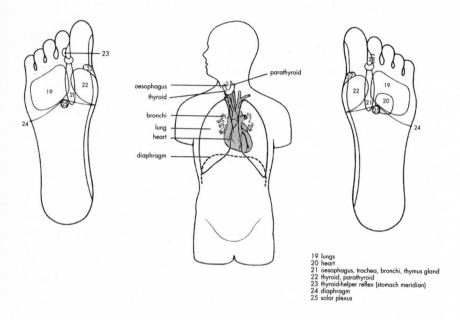

19 lungs
20 heart
21 oesophagus, trachea, bronchi, thymus gland
22 thyroid, parathyroid
23 thyroid-helper reflex (stomach meridian)
24 diaphragm
25 solar plexus

Fig. 12 The thoracic area

The oesophagus is the muscular tube passing from the pharynx down through the chest, and joining the stomach below the diaphragm. Food and fluids are propelled through it by peristalsis – wave-like contractions of the intestinal walls. The trachea passes down from the larynx into the chest where it divides into two bronchi, the main divisions of the trachea that enter the lungs.

All these reflexes are found on both feet in the same area – on the soles of the feet in a vertical band between the first and second toes.

THE THYROID GLAND

The thyroid gland is located in the neck. It produces thyroxin, which regulates the basal metabolic rate and metabolizes carbohydrates, protein and lipids. This reflex covers the entire area of the ball of the foot below the big toe, but the most important part is to be found in the half-circle shape at the base of the ball, almost under the bone of the metatarsal-phalange joint. There is also a 'helper' reflex on the second toe, where the stomach meridian is situated.

THE PARATHYROID GLANDS

These are four small glands situated around the thyroid gland. Their main function is to maintain the correct amount of calcium and phosphorus in the blood and bones. The reflex is situated on both feet at the base of the big toe on the medial side.

Meridians: The liver and spleen/pancreas meridians both begin in the big toe and end in the breast region. Both meridians have internal branches, which run through the throat area, and therefore indirectly affect the function of the throat and thyroid. The thyroid is also affected by the stomach meridian found in the second toe. Considering that the thyroid is directly involved in the metabolism of protein, carbohydrates and lipids, the quality and quantity of the wood (food) intake can be linked to many disorders of the earth element (acid/alkaline and blood sugar balances). It is interesting to note that the earth element looks after the fatty connective tissues – the roundedness of the body or the lack of. Problems in the throat, such as laryngitis or having to constantly 'clear the throat', can be directly related to a high acid level – the stomach meridian is situated on second toe. The parathyroid glands can be found on the internal section of the kidney meridian (water element). It is important to remember here the link to the hard connective tissues such as the bones, teeth and nails, as well as the balance in the body of calcium and other important minerals (see chapter 4).

THE LUNGS

The lungs are cone-shaped, spongy organs which lie in the thorax on either side of the heart. It is here that the process of respiration takes place. The air passages of the respiratory system found in the thorax are the trachea (windpipe), which divides into the bronchi to enter the left and right lungs.

The lung reflexes are found on the ball of both feet, extending from below the second toe to just past the fourth toe. Reflexes of the trachea and bronchi are found below the big toe and second toes (stomach and liver meridians) connected to the lung reflex. These same reflexes are also found in similar positions on the top of the feet.

Meridians: The stomach, kidney and gall bladder meridians all pass through sections of the lungs and all have influence on disorders of the lungs; however, very severe lung disorders, such as TB, emphysema, pneumonia and pleurisy are congestions of the internal section of the liver meridians. Again, it is interesting to note the effect of quality of wood (food) intake in relation to its oxygen and carbon dioxide levels. As when making a fire, success will depend on the quality of the wood and the air supply.

THE HEART

The heart is a hollow muscular organ, which lies in the chest on the left side of the body in a space between the lungs. It acts as a pump circulating blood throughout the body. Efficient functioning of the heart is essential to allow good blood circulation, which is necessary for efficient transport of gases, foods and waste products. The chest area also contains other major vessels leading to and from the heart – the arteries, veins, vena cavae and aorta.

The reflex to the heart is situated in the sole of the left foot only, on the kidney meridian above the diaphragm level.

THE SOLAR PLEXUS

The solar plexus is a network of sympathetic nerve ganglia in the abdomen and is the nerve supply to the abdominal organs below the diaphragm. It is sometimes referred to as the 'abdominal brain' or the 'nerve switchboard' and is situated behind the stomach and in front of the diaphragm.

The reflex is at the same level as the reflex to the diaphragm, located at a specific point in the centre of the diaphragm reflex. This point is visible on the foot as the apex of the arch that runs across the base of the ball of the foot and it is most useful for inducing a relaxed state. It can relieve stress and nervousness, aid deep regular breathing and restore calm.

Meridians: The heart reflex is positioned directly on the small internal section found on the soles of the foot starting in the fifth toe, ending in the solar plexus reflex. The main section of the kidney meridian starts from this point. In the torso, a small internal meridian also penetrates the heart, linking disorders to the kidney meridian and the water element. Looking at the control cycle of the Five Elements, we find that the water element (kidney/bladder) controls or loses control of the fire element (heart and pericardium/circulation). The pancreas meridian also has a small internal section going to the heart resulting in palpitations when losing control of the blood sugar balances. Fear, phobia and anxiety relate to the water element and are rooted in the solar plexus.

THE DIAPHRAGM

The diaphragm, one of the muscles of respiration, is a large, dome-shaped wall, which separates the thorax from the abdomen. It is the most important muscle for breathing. The reflex is situated on the soles of both feet, extends across at the base of the ball of the foot separating the ball from the arch.

Meridians: The diaphragm muscle 'belongs' to the lung meridian (see page 77), but since the muscle is penetrated by the stomach meridian, high acid levels will often result in conditions such as hiatus hernia. Considering that the lung meridian is also the metal element, this suggests that problems with the diaphragm muscle can be related to lack of minerals and vitamins, so creating an acid level.

The Abdominal Area – the Arch of the Foot

The arch of the foot is clearly visible on the sole – the raised area that extends from the base of the ball to the beginning of the heel. It is divided into two parts: the upper part corresponds to the section of the body from the diaphragm to the waistline; the lower part corresponds to the section of the body from the waistline to the pelvic area.

Reflexes above the waistline

Liver, gall bladder, stomach, pancreas, duodenum, spleen, adrenals and kidneys.

THE LIVER
The liver is the largest and most complex organ/gland in the body (other than the skin). It controls many of the chemical processes and has numerous functions. These include processing nutrients from the blood, storing fats and proteins until the body needs them, detoxifying the blood and manufacturing bile for fat digestion, storing sugars in the form of glycogen to be used when the body needs an increased supply of energy.

The reflex is found on the sole of the right foot only, below the diaphragm level, extending from the spleen/pancreas meridian on the inside of the foot to below the little toe. It ends just above the waistline.

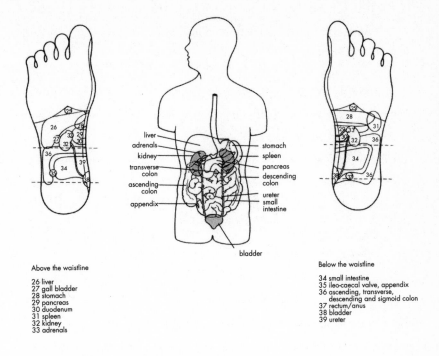

Above the waistline

26 liver
27 gall bladder
28 stomach
29 pancreas
30 duodenum
31 spleen
32 kidney
33 adrenals

Below the waistline

34 small intestine
35 ileo-caecal valve, appendix
36 ascending, transverse,
   descending and sigmoid colon
37 rectum/anus
38 bladder
39 ureter

Fig. 13 The abdominal area

THE GALL BLADDER

This is a small, muscular, pear-shaped sac attached to the under-surface of the liver; its function is to excrete bile for food digestion. The gall bladder reflex is on the sole of the right foot only, embedded within the liver reflex, beneath and between the third and fourth toes.

THE STOMACH

The stomach is a large, muscular sac that lies below the diaphragm, mainly to the left side of the body. Food passes from the mouth down the oesophagus into the stomach where it is churned up and mixed with gastric juices and enzymes to start the digestive process. The reflexes are found on the soles of both feet – extending from the big toe to the second toe on the right foot and the big toe to the outer edge of the fourth toe on the left foot. Horizontally, they are situated just below the diaphragm level.

THE PANCREAS

The pancreas is a large glandular structure in the abdomen. It is probably best known for the production of the hormones insulin and glucagons that are important in the control of sugar metabolism. The reflex is situated on the soles of both feet – more on the left foot than the right foot – below the stomach and above the waistline. On the right foot it extends to just below the big toe, and on the left foot as far as the fourth toe.

THE DUODENUM

This is the first C-shaped part of the small intestine, about 20–25 cm long. It extends from the pyloric sphincter of the stomach to the jejunum. Pancreatic and common bile ducts open into it, releasing secretions responsible for the breakdown of food. The reflexes are on the soles of both feet immediately below the pancreas, touching the waistline and extending inwards to the second toe.

THE SPLEEN

The spleen is a large, vascular, gland-like but ductless organ found on the left side of the body behind the stomach. It plays an important role in the immune system and is part of the lymphatic system. It contains lymphatic tissue which manufactures white blood cells, breaks down old red blood corpuscles and filters out toxins. The reflex is found on the outer side of the left foot (opposite the liver reflex on the right foot), beneath the fourth toe just below the diaphragm, in line with the stomach reflex.

THE KIDNEYS

The kidneys are part of the main excretory system of the body – the urinary system – which collectively comprise the kidneys, ureters, urethra and bladder. They are two bean-shaped organs, which filter toxins from the blood, produce urine and regulate the retention of important minerals and water. The reflexes are found on the soles of both feet, positioned just above the waistline on the kidney and stomach meridians, just below the stomach reflex. The right kidney is positioned slightly lower than the left kidney.

THE ADRENAL GLANDS

These are two triangular endocrine glands situated on the upper tip of each kidney. As part of the endocrine system they perform numerous vital functions. The adrenal glands are divided into two distinct regions, the cortex and medulla. The adrenal cortex produces steroid hormones, which regulate carbohydrate metabolism and have anti-allergic and anti-inflammatory properties. The cortex also produces hormones which control the re-absorption of sodium and water in the kidneys, as well as the secretion of potassium and the sex hormones testosterone, oestrogen and progesterone. The adrenal medulla produces adrenaline and noradrenaline, which work in conjunction with the sympathetic nervous system. The output of adrenaline is increased at times of anxiety and stress and is responsible for the 'fight-or-flight' reaction. The reflexes are situated on the soles of both feet on top of the kidney reflexes.

Reflexes below the waistline

Small intestine, ileo-caecal valve, appendix, large intestine, adrenals, kidneys, ureters, and bladder.

THE SMALL INTESTINE

This is a muscular tube about 6–7 m in length and is the main area of the digestive tract in which absorption takes place. It leads from the pyloric sphincter of the stomach to the caccum of the large intestine and it lies in a coiled position in the abdominal cavity surrounded by the large intestine. The small intestine is divided into three sections – the duodenum, jejunum and the ileum.

The reflex is situated on the soles of both feet, under the large intestine reflex, extending horizontally across the arch to below the fourth toe.

THE ILEO-CAECAL VALVE

This valve is situated where the small intestine and large intestine join, and therefore controls the passage of the contents of the small intestine through to the large intestine. It prevents backflow of faecal matter from the large intestine and controls mucous secretions. The reflex is found on the sole of the right foot below and between the third and fourth toes, just above the level of the pelvic floor.

THE APPENDIX

The appendix is a worm-like tube about 9–10 cm in length, with a blind end projecting downwards from the caecum of the large intestine in the lower right part of the abdominal cavity. Located directly below the ileo-caecal valve, it helps lubricate the large intestine. It is rich in lymphoid tissue and secretes antibodies. The reflex is situated on the sole of the right foot only, in the same area as the ileo-caecal valve.

THE LARGE INTESTINE

This is a tube about 1.5 m in length which surrounds the small intestine. It starts on the right side of the body at the caecum (ileo-caecal valve), goes up the right side to below the liver where it bends to the left (hepatic flexure) and passes across the abdomen as the transverse colon. At the left side of the abdomen, it bends down below the spleen (splenic flexure) to become the descending colon, which passes down the left side of the abdomen. It then turns towards the midline and takes the shapes of a double S-shaped bend known as the sigmoid flexure. This leads into the rectum, which in turn becomes the anus.

When the residue of food reaches the large intestine it is in fluid form. The function of the large intestine is to remove some of the water and salts by absorption and to convert the waste matter into faeces ready for excretion.

The reflexes are found on the soles of both feet. On the right foot this begins just below the reflex for the ileo-caecal valve and extends upwards (ascending colon), turns just below the liver reflex to become the transverse colon, which extends across the entire foot. It continues across to the left foot and turns just below the spleen reflex to become the descending colon. Just above the pelvic floor it turns again into the sigmoid colon, which ends at the reflex of the rectum/anus.

THE URETERS

The ureters are muscular tubes about 30 cm in length, which connect the kidneys and bladder, functioning as a passageway for urine. There are two tubes, one from each kidney, which pass downward through the abdomen into the pelvis where they enter the bladder. The reflexes are situated on the soles of both feet linking the kidney reflexes to the bladder reflexes, which are situated on the inner side of the instep. The ureter reflexes can often be seen as distinct lines running down the arch (following the kidney meridian).

THE BLADDER

The bladder is an elastic muscular sac situated in the centre of the pelvis. Urine for excretion passes from the kidneys down the ureters and is stored in the bladder until it is eliminated via the urethra. The reflexes are found on both feet, on the side of the foot below the inner anklebone on the heel line. This reflex is often clearly visible as a puffy area.

Meridians: When studying the pathway of the stomach meridian you will find that it is the only meridian that penetrates all the major organs of the body – hence the organs listed above, with the exception of the bladder, can be found on the stomach meridian. Other meridians, such as the spleen/pancreas, liver, gall bladder and kidney meridians, also pass through sections of some of the organs. However, an understanding of the interrelationship between the meridians and the Five Elements – with the stomach regulating the acid/alkaline balance, and the blood sugar balance regulated by its partner the spleen/pancreas meridian – will suggest an underlying cause for many of our congestions and diseases.

Finding the exact gall bladder reflex embedded in the liver reflex is possible when using the meridians. On the right foot, run your index finger up towards the ankle between the fourth and fifth toes – in the web between the metatarsals. You will find a slight indentation, which will be particularly sensitive to pressure. This is an acupuncture point on the gall bladder meridian. Once this is located, pinpoint the area directly beneath on the plantar aspect of the foot with your thumb – this will be the gall bladder reflex and for some it is embedded in the middle of the liver reflex.

The main parts of the stomach, pancreas and the duodenum will be found on the internal section of the stomach meridian, which runs almost parallel with the main section. Chronic, as well as severe disorders related to these organs can therefore be related to this division. The bladder reflex is positioned on the section of the kidney meridian found on the medial side of the foot.

The Pelvic Area – the Heel of the Foot

Few organs are represented in this section of the foot, but this area is of vital importance as all six main meridians traverse the pelvic section of the body.

THE SCIATIC NERVES

These are the largest nerves in the body. They arise from the sacral plexus of nerves formed by the lower lumbar and upper sacral spinal nerves. They run from the buttocks down the backs of the thighs to divide just above the knees into two main branches, which supply the lower legs: these are actual nerves in the feet as well as reflexes.

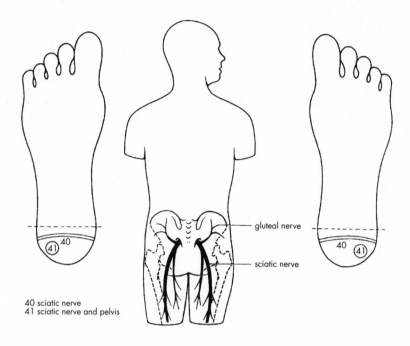

40 sciatic nerve
41 sciatic nerve and pelvis

gluteal nerve

sciatic nerve

Fig. 14 The pelvic area

The sciatic nerves and reflexes are found on the soles of both feet in a band about a third of the way down the pad of the heel extending right across the foot.

Meridians: It is interesting to note the mirror image of the sciatic nerve and the lower section of the bladder meridian. The bladder meridian also runs through the lumbar vertebrae supporting the nerve supply to these organs and nerves. Part of the actual nerve is situated in the heel. It often happens that massage to this area relieves sciatic problems.

The Reproductive Area – the Ankle

The outer ankle contains the ovaries/testes reflexes, and the inner ankle contains reflexes of the uterus, prostate, vagina and penis. The reflex points for the Fallopian tubes, lymph drainage area in the groin, vas

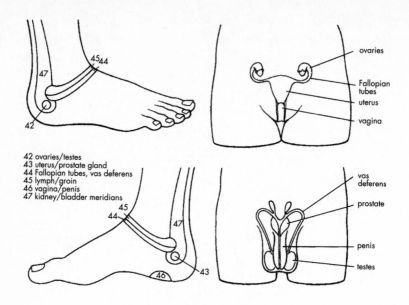

Fig. 15 The reproductive area

deferens and seminal vesicles are found in a narrow band running below the outer anklebone across the top of the foot to the inner anklebone. The kidney/bladder meridian is situated on both sides on the back of the Achilles tendon.

THE OVARIES

These are the female gonads or sex glands. They are small almond-shaped glands about 2–3 cm long. There are two ovaries – one on each side of the uterus. These are part of the female reproductive system and produce ova, as well as the hormones oestrogen and progesterone.

The reflexes are found on both feet on the lateral side, midway between the anklebone and the back of the heel – the right ovary on the right foot, the left ovary on the left foot. The 'helper' area is the heel due to the presence of the meridians.

THE TESTES

The testes are the male reproductive glands, which produce spermato-zoa and the male hormone testosterone. There are two testes suspended outside the body in the scrotum – a sac of thin dark-coloured skin, which lies behind the penis. The reflexes are found on males in the same area as the ovaries in females – midway between the lateral anklebone and the heel. The 'helper' area is the heel.

Meridians: The bladder meridian runs through this area of the foot influencing these reflexes and therefore the organs. In the body, the bladder meridian also runs through the lumbar vertebrae and the nerves supplying the reproductive organs. Furthermore, the gall bladder meridian penetrates a small section of the reflexes for the ovaries. The main section of the gall bladder meridian also penetrates the ovaries from a lateral angle and has a strong influence on the oestrogen and progesterone balance. The third meridian that penetrates the ovaries is the stomach meridian, and since sections of this meridian also traverse the face, the presence of acne may confirm assessments of congestions. In the males, the liver meridian also penetrates the testes, having an impact on the functions of the gonads.

THE UTERUS

The uterus is a hollow pear-shaped organ about 10cm long, in the centre of the pelvic cavity in females. Its function is the nourishment and protection of the foetus during pregnancy and its expulsion at term.

The reflex points are located on both feet on the medial side of the ankles, midway on a diagonal line between the ankle bone and the back of the heel. The 'helper' area is the heel.

THE PROSTATE GLAND

This gland lies at the base of the bladder in males and surrounds the urethra. It produces a thin lubricating fluid which forms part of the semen to aid the transport of sperm cells.

Reflexes are found on both feet in the same place as the uterus reflex on females – midway in a diagonal line between the medial anklebone and the heel. Again, the heel is the 'helper' area.

Meridians: The kidney meridian penetrates the uterus/prostate in the body, as well as the reflexes in the feet; according to Chinese medicine, the kidneys store the jing – a vital essence involved in reproduction. The kidney meridian also exerts an indirect effect on these organs via the internal branch meridian, which runs through the lumbar vertebrae and the nerve supply. This may suggest why many women suffer back problems during menstruation and when giving birth.

THE FALLOPIAN TUBES

In females these two tubes, about 10–14 cm in length, connect the ovaries with the cavity of the uterus. Their function is to conduct the ova expelled from the ovaries during ovulation down to the uterus.

The reflexes are found on both feet. They run across the top of the foot linking the reflex of the uterus to the reflex of the ovaries. This area is usually massaged in conjunction with the reflexes of the ovaries and uterus.

THE SEMINAL VESICLES/VAS DEFERENS

The seminal vesicles lie next to the prostate and store semen. The vas deferens is a pair of excretory ducts, which convey semen from the testes to the urethra. The reflexes are located in the same area as the Fallopian tubes in females – across the top of the foot from one ankle bone to the other, linking the prostate and testes reflexes.

Meridians: All six main meridians traverse the pelvic section of the body from different angles – however the stomach, spleen/pancreas and liver meridians will have the strongest effect on the above organs.

The Spine – the Medial Foot

The medial side of each foot is naturally curved to correspond to the spine. The spine, also known as the backbone or vertebral column, is the central support of the body. It carries the weight of the body and is an important axis of movement. The spine is made up of 33 vertebrae. The structure of the bones is arranged in such a way as to give the spine 4 curves. The spine is divided into 5 sections from top to bottom: 7 cervical vertebrae (including the axis and atlas) in the neck; 12 thoracic vertebrae in the back; 5 lumbar vertebrae in the loin; 5 sacral vertebrae in the pelvis; 4 coccygeal vertebrae in the tail. The vertebrae of the sacrum and coccyx are fused to form 2 immobile bones. Vertebrae are joined by discs of cartilage and are held in place by ligaments.

The spinal column encloses the spinal cord, the central channel of the nervous system, which is a continuation of the brain stem. It carries the nerves from the brain to all parts of the body. A pair of spinal nerves is associated with each vertebra. These nerves arise from the spinal cord and affect the level of the body at which they arise – thoracic nerves affect the thorax, lumbar nerves the lower abdomen and legs. These nerves supply specific organs so any constriction or damage to them will directly affect the connected body parts.

The spine reflex runs along the medial sides of both feet, one half of the spine being represented on each foot. The cervical vertebrae reflex runs from the base of the big toenail to the base of the toe (between the first and second joints of the big toe). The thoracic reflex runs along the ball of the foot below the big toe (shoulder to waistline), the arch from the waistline to pelvic line corresponds to the lumbar region, and the heel line to the base of the heel to the sacrum/coccyx.

Meridians: The bladder meridian is the only meridian (other than the governor vessel) that runs along the spine in the body, and therefore it has a profound effect on the spinal cord and nerves. It is the longest

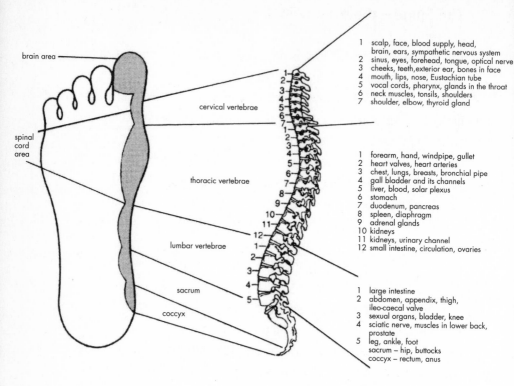

brain area

spinal cord area

cervical vertebrae

thoracic vertebrae

lumbar vertebrae

sacrum

coccyx

1 scalp, face, blood supply, head, brain, ears, sympathetic nervous system
2 sinus, eyes, forehead, tongue, optical nerve
3 cheeks, teeth, exterior ear, bones in face
4 mouth, lips, nose, Eustachian tube
5 vocal cords, pharynx, glands in the throat
6 neck muscles, tonsils, shoulders
7 shoulder, elbow, thyroid gland

1 forearm, hand, windpipe, gullet
2 heart valves, heart arteries
3 chest, lungs, breasts, bronchial pipe
4 gall bladder and its channels
5 liver, blood, solar plexus
6 stomach
7 duodenum, pancreas
8 spleen, diaphragm
9 adrenal glands
10 kidneys
11 kidneys, urinary channel
12 small intestine, circulation, ovaries

1 large intestine
2 abdomen, appendix, thigh, ileo-caecal valve
3 sexual organs, bladder, knee
4 sciatic nerve, muscles in lower back, prostate
5 leg, ankle, foot
   sacrum – hip, buttocks
   coccyx – rectum, anus

Fig. 16 The spine

meridian in the body, touches all the vertebrae and enters the brain. It therefore affects the central nervous system and, via the nerve supply, indirectly affects all the organs in the body. Taking note that a section of the meridian runs along the lateral side of the foot – in the same section as the joint reflexes – a connection to these joints should be related to the nerve supply from the spine and is influenced by the bladder meridian. Furthermore, stimulating the lateral foot directly on the bladder meridian can be of help in alleviating back problems. However, the muscles, tendons and ligaments that hold our skeletal system together and upright have a major impact on our spine. The wood element controls the tissues that give energy and strength to muscles, tendons and ligaments. High arches or flat feet are evidence of imbalances here (see page 239).

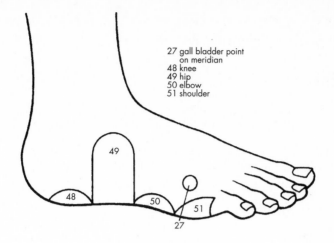

27 gall bladder point
   on meridian
48 knee
49 hip
50 elbow
51 shoulder

Fig. 17 The outer body

The Outer Body – the Lateral Foot

The lateral edge of the foot corresponds to the lateral part of the body – the joints, ligaments and surrounding muscles. From the base of the toe to the diaphragm line = shoulder and upper arm; diaphragm line to waistline = elbow, forearm, wrist and hand; waistline to end of heel = leg, knee and hip.

THE KNEE

The knee joint joins the upper and lower leg and facilitates movement of the lower limb. Reflexes are found on both feet on the outer side, just below the bony projection of the ankle bone, which is usually quite prominent on the side of the foot. Again, the six meridians run through the knee, so by pinpointing the exact location of the knee pain, one can relate it to a specific meridian and locate the problem area.

Meridians: As with the pelvic region, all six meridians penetrate the knee, but from different angles. The most common knee pains to require operations are linked with congestions found on either side of the kneecap – namely the partnership between the stomach and spleen/pancreas meridians. These knee pains are often blamed on external factors, however the acid/alkaline, as well as blood sugar balances are important aspects to include in the assessments.

THE HIP

The hip joint is where the thigh bone (femur) meets the pelvis. The reflex is found on both feet extending towards the toe in front of the knee reflex. It covers an oblong shape, moving out from the line up the side of the foot, in line with the fourth toe. A number of hip problems may be related to the gall bladder, as the gall bladder meridian passes directly through the hip.

Meridians: The gall bladder meridian is the only pathway that penetrates the hip directly from the lateral aspect of the body. You will find that the hip reflex on the foot is larger than indicated on most reflexology charts. The gall bladder meridian passes through the upper section of the reflex in line with the fourth toe; this may be puffy in look and bluish in colour, confirming that the patient is having problems with the lower back and into the hip region, and it might even show tendencies to a difference in the length of the legs. Remember that the gall bladder is part of the wood element, which governs the ligaments, tendons and the muscular system.

THE ELBOW AND SHOULDER

The elbow is the joint between the upper arm and the forearm. The humerus above and the radius and ulna below form it. The shoulder joint is where the bone of the upper arm (humerus) meets the shoulder blade (scapula).

The reflexes to the elbow are situated on both feet on the lateral side along the arch and the ball. The shoulder and the surrounding muscles are found on both feet at the base of the fifth toe covering the sole, lateral side and top.

Meridians: The lateral foot where all the joint reflexes are placed is penetrated by the bladder meridian as described above. In regards to the shoulder, a number of aspects have to be taken into consideration. The bladder meridian (fifth toe) where the shoulder reflex is found also enters the shoulder from the back of the body. Furthermore, the upper trapezius muscles in the neck belong to the kidneys. The gall bladder meridian (fourth toe) penetrates the shoulders from a lateral aspect and the anterior deltoid muscles that are used in flexing the shoulder with the elbow bent belong to the gall bladder. The lung meridian ending in the thumb penetrates the shoulder from a frontal aspect and the deltoids belong to the lungs. The small intestine meridian, ending in the little finger, penetrates the top section of the shoulder blades and stimulating the small intestine reflex might alleviate complaints here.

Three meridians, the large intestine, small intestine and triple burner penetrate the elbows from different angles and clear identification of the point of discomfort must be made in order to reach a clear assessment.

The Circulation and Breasts – the Dorsal Foot

DORSAL FOOT

Reflexes found on the dorsal section of the foot include the circulation and breasts. Here it is important to look at the meridians. If there are breast problems, note exactly where these are situated so as to identify the meridian that runs through the affected section of the breast and thereby the problem organ.

Meridians: Four meridians penetrate the sections of the breast; the very lateral section is the gall bladder, thereafter the spleen/pancreas, the stomach meridian through the nipple, and the inner section the kidney meridian. Breast problems related to each are discussed in chapter 4.

SPECIAL CIRCULATION POINTS

These points stimulate the heart, circulation and body temperature. They are situated on the dorsal and plantar of both feet at the web between the second and third toes. As these are points on the stomach meridian, they have an effect on the thyroid, which in turn affects body temperature, heart and circulation.

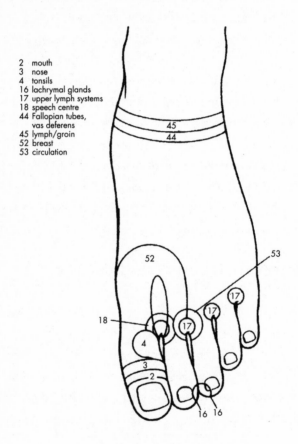

2   mouth
3   nose
4   tonsils
16 lachrymal glands
17 upper lymph systems
18 speech centre
44 Fallopian tubes,
    vas deferens
45 lymph/groin
52 breast
53 circulation

Fig. 18 The circulation and breasts

The Spiritual Mapping of the Solar Plexus

Our feet play a significant role in our spiritual well-being. They connect us to the ground and are therefore a connection between our earthly and spiritual life. They ground us both literally and figuratively. They are our base and foundation, and our contact with the earth and the energies that flow through it.

The importance of feet was recognized in Biblical times (John 13:2–10):

> 'And the supper being ended, the devil having now put into the heart of Judas Iscariot, Simon's son, to betray Him; Jesus, knowing that the Father had given all things into His hands, and that He was come from God and went to God; He riseth from supper and laid aside His garments; and took a towel and girded Himself. After that He poureth water into a basin, and began to wash His disciples' feet, and to wipe them with the towel wherewith He was girded. Then cometh he to Simon Peter; and Peter saith unto him; 'Lord dost thou wash my feet?' Jesus answered him, 'if I wash thee not thou hast no part with me.' Simon Peter saith unto Him, 'Lord, not my feet only, but also my hands and head.' Jesus saith to him, 'He that is washed needeth not save to wash his feet but is clean every whit.'

In his writings, Omraam Mikhael Aivanhov draws interesting symbolic connections between the feet and the solar plexus in relation to astrology, Christian teachings and the miracle of the five loaves and fishes.

> 'Every religion comes under the influence of two constellations diametrically opposite each other on the zodiacal circle. The Christian religion comes under the influence of Pisces (the fishes) and its polar opposite Virgo (the Virgin) and we find references to these two symbols in the Gospels.[1]

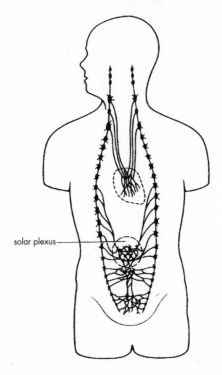

solar plexus

Fig. 19 The solar plexus and the half-moon ganglia

'Each part of our body is related to one of the constellations: Aries – head; Taurus – neck; Gemini – arms and lungs; Cancer – stomach; Leo – heart; Virgo – intestines and solar plexus; Libra – kidneys; Scorpio – genital organs; Sagittarius – thighs; Capricorn – knees; Aquarius – calves; Pisces – feet. Astrology tells us that it is the solar plexus that is in relation to Virgo and the feet to Pisces. Since Virgo and Pisces are connected and represent the axis of Christ, there must also be a connection between the feet and the solar plexus.

'The solar plexus is a part of the sympathetic nerve system which is a network of nerve fibres, ganglia and plexuses. It is located just behind the stomach and consists of five ordinary ganglia and two so-called 'half-moon' ganglia shaped like fishes. These are the five *loaves and the two fishes, the male and the female united in the solar plexus.*

'As long as a child is in its mother's womb it is bound to her by the umbilical cord through which it receives the nourishment it needs. The mother represents Nature. When a child is separated from the mother at birth the umbilical cord is cut, but there is another invisible cord which connects every child to Mother Nature who continues to nourish it. And this cord must not be cut until man is fully equipped to live his separate life, for man is a child of Nature and if the cord is cut prematurely he will no longer receive the nourishment he needs and will die. Astrology tells us that this invisible cord links man to Nature, his mother, through the solar plexus.

'The two half-moon ganglia enable man to move through space at will and the five ordinary ganglia are the five loaves with which the multitudes of his cells are nourished. Each ganglion is related to one of the five virtues symbolised by the pentagram; kindness, justice, love, wisdom and truth. The young boy who brought the loaves and fishes, which Jesus multiplied and distributed, to the multitude represents Mercury, the ruler of Virgo, in the Gospel story. And the five thousand are all the cells that make up the physical body and which receive their daily nourishment from the solar plexus.

'The loaves and fishes which were multiplied by Jesus were not ordinary material loaves and fishes ... The account of the miracle by which Jesus multiplied the loaves and fishes to feed five thousand is symbolic and should not be understood literally. In each of us the solar plexus feeds thousands upon thousands of cells with its five loaves and two fishes ... Every human being has a solar plexus, but most of them are so bogged down in material things and their lives are so chaotic that the solar plexus cannot do its

own subtle work. Every human being possesses five loaves and two fishes, but the great majority are not properly nourished; they nourish themselves on the physical plane without realising that they also need spiritual food.'[2]

Aivanhov goes on to take this theory even further.

'The Christian era was under the influence of Pisces and its opposite sign Virgo. Jesus was born of the Virgin, and he himself represents Pisces, the fish. In washing of the feet we shall once again find this Virgo–Pisces polarity, but from another point of view. 'According to the astrological tradition, there is a correspondence between man's feet and the constellation of Pisces and between the solar plexus and Virgo. If Jesus washed his disciples' feet it was in order to show them the extremely important link between the feet and the solar plexus.

'Of course it is true that with the gesture it was as though Jesus was telling his disciples, "This is an example I am giving you. Later on you too will have to show the same humility and unselfishness towards others." And he then washed Judas' feet although he knew perfectly well that Judas had already betrayed him. Symbolically you could say that someone who refuses to take revenge on those who have done him a wrong washes their feet. But Jesus' gesture was, above all, intended to awaken in his disciples the constructive energies of the solar plexus. The seven main Chakras repeat themselves in reverse order from the coccyx down to the feet. With this esoteric theory the Crown Chakra is represented on the soles of the feet. The Christ washed the disciples' feet in order to awaken the Crown Chakra above the head, to awaken the spiritual energies.

'Probably in the ordinary circumstances of daily life, some of you have already noticed a connection between your feet and your

solar plexus. When your feet are cold you can feel a tightening of the solar plexus, and if you eat while you're feeling like that, your digestion will be more difficult than usual. But you will find that if you soak your feet in hot water it will give you a delightful sensation of relaxation at the level of your solar plexus and you will feel on top of your form. That is why, if you are feeling anxious or tense, I advise you to consciously and deliberately prepare a basin of hot water, to soak your feet in it and wash them with attention: in this way you will be influencing and strengthening your solar plexus and your state of consciousness will immediately be transformed ...

'We must never forget that it is by means of our feet that we maintain the contact with the earth and its telluric currents: they serve as antennae. But the electro-magnetic currents arising from the earth or flowing down into it can only circulate freely if the feet are not charged with layers of fluidic impurities; that is why it is good to wash one's feet every evening.

'To begin with Peter refused to let Jesus wash his feet and later he asked him to wash not only his feet but his head and hands as well, and Jesus told him: "He that is washed needeth not save to wash his feet, but is clean every whit." The feet being the part of the body which is most closely in contact with the earth, they represent the physical plane which we have to transcend in order to gain access to higher planes, and this is why if we consciously fix our attention on and under our feet while we are washing them, we can work towards this liberation from the physical plane ...

'The feet therefore symbolise the physical sphere and of course it is in the physical sphere that we are always victimised since the feet symbolise the most material, to wash one's feet represents the final touch in the work of purification ...

'So, as you can see, Jesus' gesture in washing his disciples' feet has a much deeper significance than is usually realised ... Begin to work on your feet and your solar plexus on a spiritual level and you will soon feel very beneficial results.'[3]

The Vacuflex System

Lastly, a further interesting technique for mapping the feet is by means of the Vacuflex system of diagnosis and treatment. This is described in detail in the Appendix at the end of the book (see pages 304–7).

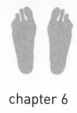

chapter 6

anatomy, structure and conditions of the feet

But is it not sweet with nimble feet
To dance upon the air!

OSCAR WILDE

The Anatomy of the Foot

The human foot is an architectural masterpiece. Although the foot is a fraction of the size of the body, it balances, supports and transports the entire body weight. The structure of the foot forms the base and the anchorage point for the upright position of a human being. A stable anchorage point relies on correct alignment and joint function of the foot and lower limb, and any impairment can displace the centre of gravity. When this occurs, other parts of the body will compensate and this can result in knee, leg and calf pains and also in back problems.

Some people view the human body as a machine and think it acceptable to misuse it, since it can always be fixed, a spare part sewn on or patched in, or, if a bodily system breaks down, that drugs will be able to fix it. When we operate from a fix-all mentality, we tend to negate the interconnectedness of the human being, the wholeness of the human organism – the fact that man is body, mind and spirit. According to the medical professions, the structure of the foot can be damaged severely by ill-fitting shoes, incorrect posture and being involved in activities that produce excessive stress, such as running and ballet. These activities can cause foot deformities ranging from corns and calluses to more serious damage such as bunions and enlarged toe joints.

Foot deformities and irregularities can also affect the reflexes and meridians on which they manifest. This, in turn, can affect the corresponding body parts by causing congestion in energy flow, thus possibly affecting associated organs.

The Bones of the Feet

Bones provide a framework and the supporting structure for many of the body's tissues. The foot is divided into three groups: 14 phalanges at the anterior of the foot that constitute the toes; 5 metatarsals and 2 sesamoids in the middle of the foot that together make up the instep.

At the posterior of the foot there are 7 bones; a navicular bone, 3 cuneiform bones, a cuboid bone, the talus or anklebone and the calcaneus or heel bone. The 2 main weight-bearing bones of the foot are the calcaneus, the heel bone, with the talus or anklebone resting directly upon it. The navicular transmits weight to the cuneiform bones and in turn they transmit weight to the first metatarsal bones, which then carry the weight.

Next to the navicular is the cuboid that receives the weight transmitted forward by the calcaneus and transmits it to the fourth and fifth metatarsal bones. The five metatarsal bones transmit weight to the forward part of the foot.

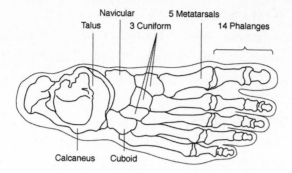

Fig. 1 Bones of the foot

Under the head of the metatarsal bones are the two small sesamoid bones located independently of the skeleton system, since they do not join with any other bones. They act to protect the tendon as it moves back and forth.

The main function of the phalanges of the toes that join with the metatarsals is to give spring to the step.

Four arches of the feet

The inner longitudinal arch acts like a spring, absorbing the natural shocks that come from walking. The calcaneus, the talus, the cuneiform bones and the three inner metatarsals form the arch. The 28 bones in the foot bear the entire weight of the body on four arches. The arches give feet their shape. Two of the arches run across the foot, while the other two run the length of the foot. Generally, the arches 'give' or stretch slightly when weight is applied to the foot, and spring back when the weight is removed.

TRANSVERSE ARCH

The transverse arch is formed by the cuboid and the three cuneiform bones. As a person's weight comes down, it is accepted by the transverse arch.

ANTERIOR METATARSAL ARCH

The anterior metatarsal arch is formed at the point where the metatarsal bones join the phalanges and it runs across the foot. This arch flattens out when the front ends of the metatarsals bear weight.

MEDIAL LONGITUDINAL ARCH

The medial (inner) longitudinal arch is formed by the calcaneus, talus, cuneiforms and the three inner metatarsals and it runs the length of the inside of the foot. It acts like a spring, absorbing the natural impacts that come from walking.

LATERAL LONGITUDINAL ARCH

The lateral longitudinal arch is formed by the calcaneus, the cuboid and the fourth and fifth metatarsals. The lateral (outer) arch (solid and flat), receives and carries the greatest part of the body weight.

Foot joints

Joints are formed whenever two bones meet. The 33 complex joints in each foot permit great flexibility of movement. The ends of the bones are covered with cartilage, a soft, smooth substance, and they are lubricated by synovial fluid. The bones are held together with elastic fibrous ligaments. The joints come in two types.

HINGE JOINT

This allows extension and flexion (bending up and down and to move forwards and backwards). The ankle and toe joints are typical hinge joints.

PLANE JOINT

A flat surface that allows the bones, such as the tarsals and metatarsals, to slide on each other, but ligaments restrict this movement to a small range.

Muscles, tendons and ligaments of the foot

Muscles provide the power needed to move the feet and toes. When a muscle contracts, it pulls on a tendon, which in turn moves the bone. Muscles become painful if overused or deprived of oxygen due to poor circulation.

Tendons, which attach muscles to bones, can also become painful when damaged by stresses similar to those that cause torn ligaments – the large tendon at the heel, the Achilles tendon, is a common site for such problems.

The calf muscles are very important for their pumping action, which squeezes the blood in the veins back to the heart, allowing fresh oxygenated blood to flow into the leg and foot.

Muscles that move the ankle, foot and toes

Muscles located in the lower limb work together to move the ankle, foot and toes. Moving the foot upwards is termed 'dorsal flexion'; downwards is termed 'plantar flexion'. Turning the sole of the foot inwards is termed 'inversion'; outwards is termed 'eversion'. Muscles attach the femur, tibia and fibula to bones of the feet and enable the feet to perform certain movements.

DORSAL FLEXORS
The tibialis anterior moves the foot upwards and inwards; peroneus tertius moves the foot upwards and outwards and extensor digitorum longus moves the foot upwards and moves the foot and toes outwards.

PLANTAR FLEXORS
The gastrocnemius moves the foot downwards and soleus moves the foot downwards

Nails

Nails protect the tips of the toes from abnormal pressure or rubbing. They are hard, horny and colourless protective plates, which grow usually in a straight line from the nail root. If injury to the root interrupts the nail's natural protective growth pattern, the toenail will then grow either abnormally thick or to one side.

Bone and Joint Disorders

Bunion (hallux valgus)

Bunion or hallux valgus is a condition in which the side of the big toe joint (the metatarso-phalangeal joint) becomes painful and enlarged. The big toe moves sideways towards the middle of the foot, which means that the joint is no longer articulating in a normal manner. As hallux valgus progresses, the tendons of the toes shorten, the muscles contract and all the bones of the foot are displaced. The bunion presses against the shoe, irritating the skin and causing pain.

The big toe's movement towards the middle of the foot is very often accompanied by the little toe's movement towards the middle of the foot. This results in a 'bunion' on the outer side of the foot over the fifth metatarso-phalangeal joint and is often referred to as a 'bunionette'.

A different type of bunion is caused by bursitis, which is an inflammation of a bursa. The bursa is a sac containing tissue fluid which acts as a lubricant between the skin and the bones at the big toe joint. Continual irritation of the skin causes the sac to become inflamed and inflated with fluid. When that occurs, the condition is an acute and painful bursitis.

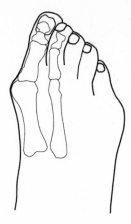

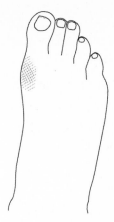

Fig. 2a Bunions   *Fig. 2b Bursitis*

THE CAUSES ACCORDING TO WESTERN MEDICAL THEORY

Continued wearing of pointed shoes or displacement of foot due to high-heeled shoes; inherited joint weakness and injury or inflammation in the joint.

TREATMENT

Prescription shoes with a wider forefoot, surgery – called a bunionectomy – or cortisone injections for pain relief.

SELF-TREATMENT

Use shoes that don't cramp your bunion or protective pads to ease discomfort.

Hammertoes

This condition often accompanies bunions, as this affliction is most common on the second toe. It is produced by a muscle imbalance, which causes the distal joints of the toes to bend backwards. The medial joints bend so that the toe rises above the other toes and the distal joint is almost curled underneath. Joints may stiffen permanently. When hooked toes rub and chaff against the shoes, painful corns and calluses develop.

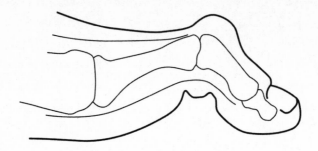

Fig. 3 Hammetoe

THE CAUSES ACCORDING TO WESTERN MEDICAL THEORY
Similar to the causes which produce bunions; shoes aggravate this condition. Constriction of the foot into narrow shoes can cause foot muscles to waste away by depriving them of movement. High-arched feet are more inclined to develop hammertoes because of the positioning of the ligaments pulling on the toes.

TREATMENT
With age, hammertoes may become rigid and require surgery to correct.

Rigid toe (hallux rigidus)

The big toe fuses with the metatarsal bone and creates unnatural stiffness. The toe loses its flexibility and walking is hampered.

THE CAUSES ACCORDING TO WESTERN MEDICAL THEORY
A rigid toe can be the result of osteoarthritis, injury, obesity and flat feet.

TREATMENT
As flexibility decreases, movement is curtailed. Joint replacement is a solution to this problem.

Swollen painful joints

THE CAUSES ACCORDING TO WESTERN MEDICAL THEORY

Arthritis and gout are often responsible for swollen painful joints. If this condition becomes chronic, it can lead to deformity and immobility of the person.

Arthritis causes cartilage to degenerate; the bones either become enlarged or waste away. As the linings of the joints become stiff, painful and swollen, the muscles that move the joints are unable to function and waste away. Two types of arthritis usually occur – osteoarthritis, which is a degenerative condition attacking the cartilage around the bone ends, and rheumatoid arthritis, which is a chronic inflammation of the joints. It is progressive and incapacitating.

Gout usually attacks the big toe joint. It is caused by an excess of uric acid in the blood. It causes painful inflammation and swelling of the joints of the toes. The person may feel ill and run a fever. It is an acute condition and medical intervention is often required.

TREATMENT

The factors that are causing the swollen painful joints are usually addressed. If the conditions are acute, medical intervention is required. Chronic conditions can be controlled by means of nutritional advice and a lifestyle change, incorporating a change to a more alkaline diet and a constant physical exercise regime.

The link to the meridians and the five elements

BONES/JOINT DISORDERS

The skeleton system, and therefore the bones, are a division of the body's hard connective tissues, which together with the tissues of the nails and teeth, is linked to the water element in traditional Chinese medicine

(TCM). Any weakness with the Chi in the water element and its meridians – the bladder and kidney – can manifest into frail bones and other bone and joint disorders. It is interesting to note that the internal section of the kidney meridian goes through the parathyroid (see page 136), therefore the link to the hard connective tissues becomes understandable. Many of these disorders are also linked to high acid levels, so when assessing patients it will be useful to keep in mind that the earth element – controlling your acid and alkaline balance – controls or loses control over the water element.

BUNIONS
Bunions manifest on the spleen/pancreas meridian and the thyroid reflex (see chapter 4, page 102).

HAMMERTOES
Hammertoes mostly manifest on the second and third toes linking the condition to the stomach meridian (see chapter 4, page 97). However, any of the toes can show evidence of the tendons and ligaments becoming shorter and therefore bending. The wood element controls the strength or weakness of the tissues of tendons, ligaments and muscles; it also represents the quality of food intake, and controls or loses control of the acid/alkaline, as well as blood sugar levels.

GOUT
Gout, a uric acid condition, usually attacks the big toe; however TCM links the condition to the liver meridian; the same goes for rigid toe (see chapter 4, page 158).

Skin disorders

Athlete's foot

Athlete's foot is a fungal infection that usually starts in the warm, moist areas between the toes, especially the fourth and fifth toes. The most obvious sign of infection is an edge of scaly, loose skin forming a ring around an area of pink, itchy skin and tiny blisters. An area of white soggy water-laden skin often accompanies the fungus.

A fungus does not create a disease. It is most likely a parasite, which grows on live tissue and must have a proper medium to feed on, such as the skin. Conditions favourable to fungus growth are encouraged by our lifestyle patterns. In particular, sugar, yeasts, and antibiotics in our diet allow fungi to thrive.

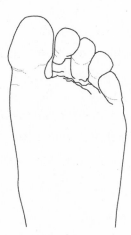

Fig. 4 Athlete's foot

THE CAUSES ACCORDING TO WESTERN MEDICAL THEORY
Several factors increase vulnerability to a fungus infection such as inadequate ventilation of the feet due to closed plastic shoes. Excessive perspiration can cause maceration of the feet. Allergic reaction to sweat, drugs and dyes. Going barefoot in public baths, showers and swimming pools. Not drying adequately between toes after bathing or

showering. Impaired circulation. The perspiration of a diabetic is rich in sugar, making it a perfect medium for fungi to thrive in. Contaminated articles of clothing, such as shoes, slippers, stockings or those for personal use like towels and bathmats.

TREATMENT
Anti-fungal powders, ointments, cream and spray obtained from chemist and antibiotics.

SELF-TREATMENT
Use tea tree oil or apple cider vinegar; follow a healthy nutritional lifestyle.

Corns and calluses

Corn and calluses are concentrated areas of hard skin, with no roots or living parts. The corn is usually found over a prominent and fixed joint of a toe. The nucleus of hard skin in the centre of the corn presses on nearby nerve endings to produce the stabbing pain of the corn. Calluses are found on the sole of the foot in an area that is receiving an excessive amount of pressure and friction. Initially, this hard skin is protective and in many cases is painless and trouble-free. The build-up of a callus may go beyond that required for protection and can lead to pain and discomfort.

THE CAUSES ACCORDING TO WESTERN MEDICAL THEORY
A poorly styled or badly fitted shoe combined with the shape and position of the foot and toes is usually the cause of friction taking place on the skin. High-heeled shoes are a major cause of calluses developing on the balls of the feet. Calluses can also arise from chronic skin conditions such as eczema (see below), fungus infections, stretched ligaments in the foot and thyroid malfunction. Poor blood circulation and diabetes can each turn an ordinary callus into a deep weeping ulcer.

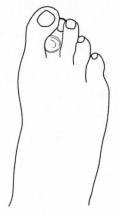
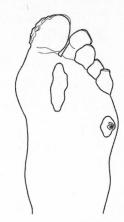

Fig. 5 Corn on second toe   *Fig. 6 Callus on oesophagus reflex*

TREATMENT

Removal of the callus by the chiropodist. An insole or a device to improve the position and functioning of the foot or protective pad to ease discomfort.

SELF TREATMENT

Soak the foot in a solution of bicarbonate of soda – when the callus has softened sufficiently, the thickened skin can be rubbed away with a pumice stone. Make sure properly fitted footwear is worn.

Plantar wart (verruca plantaris)

A plantar wart is a raised lump of flesh on the sole of the foot. They can also occur on the toes or the top of the foot. It is pearly white, soft and spongy, with a centre that shows tiny spots of black, brown or red. When pinched slightly it causes an excruciating pain, indicating it is a plantar wart. Plantar warts can grow either singly or in clusters.

THE CAUSES ACCORDING TO WESTERN MEDICAL THEORY

Medical science shows evidence that they are caused by a virus. All warts are spread by scratching or shaving, or by going barefoot in public places.

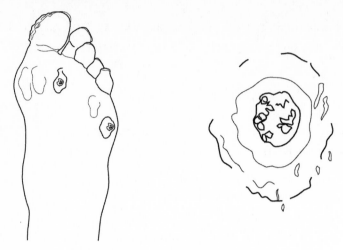

Fig. 7 Verruca plantaris *(plantar warts)*

TREATMENT

Cauterising the warts with acid, laser surgery or freezing them with dry ice. Vitamin A has been prescribed.

Eczema

This is an acute or chronic inflammatory condition of the skin of the feet. Skin eczema can occur as papules, which become moist and finally form scabs. Dry eczema also occurs as dry scaly areas on the foot, especially on top of the foot and toes. The causes and treatment are the same as for athlete's foot (see pages 231–2).

Disorders associated with the heel of the foot

The heel bears the downward impact of the body weight when walking, and is subject to immense stress. The calcaneus is the largest bone in the foot with a protective layer of fatty tissue. Certain disorders do, however, develop.

HEEL CALLUS

This is formed when the skin around the edge of the heel becomes thicker than usual to protect it from external pressure and friction.

HEEL FISSURES

These develop when the skin on the edge of the heel splits. This can result from the skin being excessively dry, from wearing incorrectly fitted shoes or walking barefoot over harsh terrain. If the fissures are deep, bleeding can occur and the area can become infected.

HEEL SPUR

This is a bony growth on the underside of the heel bone and can cause pain on the bottom of the heel when standing. Overweight people often develop heel spurs. These spurs are the results of a torn longitudinal ligament that bleeds, generating fibrous tissue which ultimately calcifies. Heel spurs can become inflamed and painful.

The link to the meridians and the five elements

SKIN DISORDERS

As the protective layer of our body, skin gets its strength from the metal element that controls the tissues of our skin. Regardless of the condition of the skin – whether it is oily or dry – disorders such as eczema, corns and calluses all communicate the state of Chi within the metal element and the lung and colon meridians. As we have seen, the metal element can represent the quality and quantity of vitamins, minerals and enzymes obtained from our food. In order to accurately assess a skin condition, it is essential to ascertain exactly where on the foot or body it occurs, and thus on which meridian or reflex it lies. It is interesting to note that many skin conditions exhibit symmetry on the body – for instance, if eczema or dry skin is found on the one elbow or buttock, it is consistently found parallel on the other side. This is due to the meridians being in pairs mirroring each other.

ATHLETE'S FOOT

Athlete's foot is mostly found between the fourth and fifth toes representing the bladder and kidney meridians (see Chapter 4, page 131).

CORNS

Corns can be found on the top or side of any of the toes; however, many case studies show corns on the second toe (stomach meridian) or the fourth toe (gall bladder meridian (see Chapter 4, page 152).

CALLUSES

Calluses can be found on many places on the feet; they are commonly on the ball of the foot, indicating a weakness within the respiratory system and the metal element. Calluses, dry or cracked (fissures) in the heel have to be related to the pelvic area of the body. However, on the medial aspect of the foot notice should be taken of the spleen/pancreas meridian and the fact that it penetrates the pelvic organs. Many females present a cracked, dry callus on the medial side of the heel when experiencing menstrual problems; similarly with men experiencing prostate problems. The lateral side of the heel is related to the gall bladder meridian, and a dry, cracked heel is often a sign that there might be hip pain or lower back into the hip complaints (see chapter 4, page 152).

ECZEMA

Like any other skin condition, eczema relates to metal imbalances. It is interesting to note the relationship to the colon and/or lung problems that many sufferers report. Many children start with asthma/allergy and later suffer from eczema (or vice versa), the first condition having been treated medically with antibiotics that suppressed the condition rather than correcting the imbalances. Whether someone suffers from a colon condition, respiratory problems or a skin condition, they will be confirming a low state of Chi within the metal element. This will indicate a need to take a better look at the quality of their food intake, and the possibility of the use of supplements.

HEEL SPUR

Heel spur is bony growth related to the hard connective tissues that are governed by the water element and its meridians, the bladder and kidney.

Toenail disorders

INGROWN TOENAIL

This is a common and painful condition. It usually occurs on the big toe when the side of the nail penetrates the skin of the nail groove and becomes embedded in the soft skin tissue. Incorrect cutting of the toenail – either cutting the nail too short or cutting down the sides – can cause this problem.

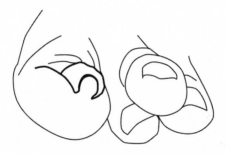

Fig. 8a Ingrown toenail

THICKENED TOENAIL

The thickening of the toenail occurs when the nail cell production is damaged. This occurs when the toenail has sustained an injury or if the toenail is persistently rubbing against a shoe. The nail becomes extremely hard and very difficult to pedicure. The nail growth often curves over the edge to form a 'ram's-horn' nail, which is both unsightly and uncomfortable. Many elderly people suffer from this condition.

FUNGAL INFECTION

This painful and uncomfortable condition is termed onychomycosis and in acute situations the toenails have to be removed. The fungus penetrates the toenail and causes it to thicken and appear dry, lustre-less, scaly and streaked. Often it has a grey, yellow or brown colouring, which can affect the whole nail or only the part where the nail is affected. Medical treatment should be sought.

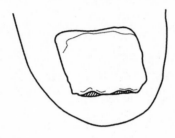

Fig. 8b Fungal nail

The link to the meridians and the five elements

NAIL CONDITIONS

Within TCM, there are two elements involved in regard to the appear-ance of the nails. The hard connective tissues – those that build and give strength to the nails – obtain Chi from the water element. Condi-tions showing imbalances are soft, peeling and split nails which are mainly found on the fingernails. It is important to take note which fin-ger or toenail is showing weakness. However, when it comes to the look of the nails, this relates to the wood element and can be evidence of foodstuffs that are stressing the system (see chapter 4, page 151).

INGROWN TOENAIL

Most ingrown toenails happen in the big toe. The medial side of the nail relates to the spleen/pancreas meridian and the lateral side the liver meridian (see chapter 4, page 165). It is interesting to note that it is often the younger and older generations that suffer most from this condition. It is possible that we need to observe that both the younger and elder person are prone to having deficiencies in their food intake due to their lifestyles.

Disorders affecting the arches of the foot

FLAT FEET (PES PLANUS)

Flat feet are caused by a muscle imbalance. Although the condition can be genetically inherited, it can also be developed due to a weakness in the joints, overweight or as a result of long illness. This results in flattened arches with the whole foot making contact with the ground. The condition can bring about hammertoes, bunions, fatigue of the arches, pain in the whole foot, lower limb and, especially, in the calf region.

HIGH-ARCHED FEET (PES CAVUS)

A high-arched foot is usually stiff and rigid – this limits manoeuvrability of the foot and prevents efficient functioning of the foot. This is commonly a genetically inherited condition. A problem encountered with this condition refers to incorrect weight bearing of the foot. Because of the pitch of the foot, the weight is transferred to the head of the metatarsal. This can result in tired, aching feet and heels, and ankle pain with corns and calluses developing on the toe joints as the toes assume a 'claw foot' position.

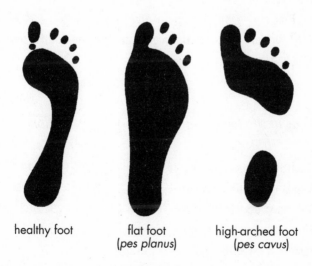

healthy foot   flat foot   high-arched foot
                      (*pes planus*)   (*pes cavus*)

Fig. 9 Flat feet and high-arched feet

METATARSALGIA

This is pain in the ball of the foot resulting from a rigid high-arched foot or from spreading of the lower foot with age.

PLANTAR NEUROMA

This is nerve growth that often accompanies metatarsalgia. It develops when the nerve between two metatarsal heads, especially between the third and fourth toes, is pinched. This results in numbness.

PLANTAR FASCIITIS

This is a chronic inflammation of the plantar fascia, a ligament-like structure that passes from the heel to the forefoot. The fascia partially pulling away from the heel causes the inflammation.

The link to the meridians and the five elements

MUSCLES, TENDONS AND LIGAMENTS OF THE FOOT (OR ANY PART OF THE BODY)

The wood element governs the strength of these tissues, hence any condition that changes the shape of the foot or body has to be related to stress to the gall bladder and liver, and their meridians (see chapter 4, pages 152, 155).

Conditions in the feet resulting from poor circulation

Poor circulation can affect the feet. As they are furthest from the heart, they are prone to suffer from inadequate circulation. Cramps, numbness, varicose veins and infection are symptoms of poor circulation.

RAYNAUD'S DISEASE

This is a condition that affects the arteries in the fingers and toes, making the fingers and toes go noticeably white when first reacting to the cold and, later, as they return to normal, go through a period when they are coloured blue and then bright red, at which stage they are painful. In some people, the shut-off of the blood vessels causes problems to the tissues, especially in the toes, causing them to become shortened and tapered in appearance.

Foot Care for Diabetics

The blood vessels that carry blood to the leg and foot can become reduced in diameter, so reducing the amount of blood circulating. Without a good and adequate supply of blood, valuable nutrients, oxygen and the white blood cells, which provide our defence against infection, will be in short supply.

CONDITIONS RESULTING FROM DIABETES MELLITUS

Loss of sensation in the feet due to damage to the nerve endings. Brittle cracked skin and danger of cuts or sores developing into ulceration or gangrene. Poor circulation/reduced blood flow, oedema (swelling), excessive sweating and loss of elasticity of skin.

The link to the meridians and the five elements

BLOOD AND CIRCULATION

Labels such as 'hardening of the arteries', 'varicose veins', and 'cold hands and feet', all refer to symptoms confirming a lack of Chi in the fire element. The Chi of the fire element is what gives us the zest for life and the best of health; hence the lack of fire or a bad quality of fire will have a major impact on our life profile. Any of the diseases related to a fire imbalance show the ultimate quality of our food intake. Our food can be the best medicine or the worst poison.

Foot Care

It pays to take care of your feet. Time and attention not only keeps your feet looking and feeling good, but will have further health benefits. Having now assessed that every part of the foot represents a part of the body, the relevance of treating the feet with care and kindness is obvious. Good hygiene is of primary importance. Foot hygiene focuses on washing the feet thoroughly every day to remove dead skin and eliminate bacteria. The average foot gives off about half a cup of moisture a day. The skin becomes soft and soggy as a result of the moisture, making it easier for friction to cause blisters, for chemicals to leach from shoes and cause contact dermatitis, and for athlete's foot and other forms of fungi to take hold. The most common problem from all this moisture is bromhidrosis – a scientific term for smelly feet. This occurs because the foot's warmth and sweat provide choice growing conditions for bacteria. Paying special attention to the type of footwear you use can also reduce perspiration. But most of all take note of the relationship to the meridians and therefore your lifestyle.

There are a few basic foot-care hints that all of us should follow:

- Wash your feet carefully and dry thoroughly, especially between the toes;
- Allow your feet to 'air out' – don't keep them locked up in shoes all the time;
- Trim you toenails straight across;
- Use creams to keep the skin supple and powders on your feet to absorb extra moisture and prevent making an environment for infections and bacteria to grow and odour to manifest;
- Regular pedicures are very beneficial;
- Wear socks and shoes that fit properly;
- Rest your feet during the day;
- Be kind to your feet, do not abuse them.

Regular washing and careful drying will help prevent cracks developing. A pumice stone and creams will help soften hardened areas. Problems such as corns, verrucas and athlete's foot should be attended to, and a chiropodist consulted for persistent problems. Feet should also be kept warm and comfortable during colder days. Changes in foot temperature can exacerbate health problems (see chapter 4, page 142).

Feet treats – footbaths

Herbalist and healer Maurice Messegue recommended herbal footbaths as an essential part of his treatment. He believed treatment by osmosis to be most effective since the main healing ingredients rapidly penetrate the skin and may reach the affected areas faster than if the same ingredients are taken internally. He chose foot and hand baths over hip and full baths as they are easy to prepare and because the hands and feet are the most receptive parts of the body. Baths can be prepared with dried herbs or aromatherapy oils infused in boiling water. Footbaths should be taken as hot as possible, first thing in the morning on an empty stomach, and should not last for more than eight minutes.

Most people are born with healthy feet – it is estimated that about 80% of adults develop self-induced foot disorders. 'My feet are killing me' is a common expression used in reference to sore feet at the end of a day, but it holds a great deal of truth and can reveal a deeper insight into the body. The body is trying to communicate to us that there is a state of internal deterioration. It is the body's cry for help, to call our attention to the harm that we are imposing on our bodies – do not disregard sore feet.

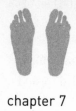

chapter 7

the treatment sequence

'Those who are habitually without disease help to train and to adjust those who are sick, for those who treat should be free from illness. They train the patient to adjust his breathing and in order to train the patient, they act as examples.'

NEI CHING

The Responsibilities of a Reflexologist

The most important asset a therapeutic reflexologist can have is genuine compassion for the suffering of humanity and a desire to assist in relieving this suffering. But if you intend to become a practising reflexologist, you must approach your task with complete and utter professionalism. A thorough knowledge of the subject – reflexes, TCM, foot structure, as well as good basic knowledge of anatomy, physiology, pathology and patho-physiology – will increase your competence.

A clean, hygienic workspace or clinic is necessary to create the correct impression. Everything about the reflexologist should give the impression of professionalism – the surroundings, your attire and approach. To quote from the Nei Ching:

'Poor medical workmanship is neglectful and careless and must therefore be combated, because a disease that is not completely cured can easily breed new disease or there can be a relapse of the old disease ... The most important requirement of the art of healing is that no mistakes or neglect occur.'

Make sure the patient understands the reflexology procedure. A thorough knowledge of the subject will give the patient confidence in your ability to facilitate in the healing process. Reflexology, as a pressure-technique practised mainly on the feet, is an intimate treatment and the patient must be made to feel comfortable. The patient will often feel the need to talk, and this should be encouraged. Healing, apart from the scientific aspect, is an art which requires intuitive skills. The art of assessing the roots of patients' problems and working with them to overcome these problems can only be learnt through experience, practise, self-knowledge and constant attentiveness to the individual patient.

Preparing for a Reflexology Treatment

Before a patient arrives, you should prepare the treatment room and ensure that all materials and supplies you may need are available and within reach. Check that your equipment, such as your therapy couch/bed and therapist chair is in good working order, and that you have a safe disposal facility for used materials. The most effective therapist chairs are small round chairs on wheels, which allow you to swivel from side to side and can be adjusted to a comfortable working height. It is preferable not to use chairs with arm rests as these can be cumbersome and prevent you from getting into the right sitting position when performing the treatment.

Hygiene plays an important role in any therapy room – check that your room and equipment are clean and that you have fresh towels and linen. Most therapists keep a supply of cotton wool, disinfectants, herbal creams/oils, and pen and paper in their therapy rooms. Be sure to check that you have enough stock on hand for the duration of the treatment.

A reflexology treatment should be a pleasurable experience. Many people may feel apprehensive at the prospect of their first reflexology treatment, so it is your responsibility to ensure that the patient is made to feel welcome and comfortable. Always be caring and compassionate and reassure the patient that they are in good hands. As relaxation is of prime importance in the healing process, the surroundings must be as peaceful and organized as possible. Once the session has begun, all distractions must be avoided. Interruptions will not assist in achieving the desired effect.

People have strange attitudes regarding their feet and many will be embarrassed about their state. Any insecurities of this type must be dispelled. Feet are a reflexologist's domain – they specialize in feet and are accustomed to seeing them in all shapes, sizes and conditions. The feet represent the body and encompass a wealth of information about one's state of health. They are the key to revealing where imbalances lie and play a vital role in the enhancement of general health and well-being.

Medical Case History

At the first treatment, the therapist begins by taking a thorough medical case history. All problems must be noted, not just those troubling the patient at the time. This detail is necessary as all problems are relevant in ascertaining a complete health picture.

In order to understand the patient's complaint, it is advisable to record a detailed case history. This is used for reference during ensuing treatments to gauge progress. Details that should be recorded include current medical complaints, past symptoms and illnesses, previous operations, allergies and intolerances, family history, current and previous medication. Other pertinent details include dietary habits and general lifestyle (past and present), as well as more emotional issues such as the patient's motivations and goals in life, management of their current lifestyle, such as stress management. Obviously, you can develop your own case history form to suit your individual requirements.

Guidelines for compiling a case history

Firstly, note the complaint for which treatment is being sought. Then take note of all other symptoms and treatments in as much detail as possible. If headaches are a symptom, note where these occur – forehead, neck tension and the like – in order to trace them to a specific meridian. If they occur on the bladder meridian, check whether the patient has a history of bladder problems. If they occur on the gall bladder meridian, other symptoms may include nausea or intolerance of fatty foods, and thus a gall bladder imbalance may be pin-pointed as the cause.

Check thoroughly through each body system, questioning the functions – digestion, bowels, bladder and blood pressure. Does the patient feel mentally alert? How do they cope with stress? Is their energy level depleted? Do they suffer from heartburn or other digestive disorders? What exercise do they take? Observe the skin, hair and nail condition and record this. What of the endocrine system? If female, record all problems related to the menstrual cycle – regular, painful, heavy or long menstruation, and pre-menstrual tension symptoms. If male, record any problems with their prostate. Also record all previous treatment. In this way one can determine which meridians dominate the problems. It is necessary to ask personal questions which may embarrass some patients, but they should be reassured. Question them on how long the problem took to develop, how long it has been present, accompanying aches and pains, eating and drinking habits, parents' eating habits, and hereditary tendencies.

It is interesting to observe family history and inherited problems and note how these manifest in related complaints. Often diseases have the same root cause and are situated along the same meridians, but the symptoms may differ. For example, you may be treating a mother and she decides to bring her child. The mother may suffer breast problems and painful ovaries, while the child suffers from acne and chest weakness – all of which symptoms manifest along the stomach meridian. Dietary indiscretions can often be cited as the main culprit of hereditary weaknesses.

It is not wise to force dietary change on patients, but one should try and enlighten them regarding dietary related problems and help steer them towards a more healthy way of eating. Using the stomach meridian as an example, point out to the patient problems which can arise from dietary indiscretions. Once they understand the cause of pain and discomfort, they will be more willing to change their ways.

Keep a comprehensive record of each treatment, checking all reactions, both good and bad, as well as changes in general health. At the same time, you should record the lifestyle advice you have given your patient during or after the treatment, as well as any recommendations or referrals made.

Reflexologists Don't ...

Reflexologists don't practise medicine. That is the realm of orthodox licensed physicians. Reflexologists never diagnose a disease, treat a specific condition, prescribe or adjust medication. They do not treat specific diseases, although reflexology helps eliminate problems caused by these diseases. By bringing the body back into a state of balance, reflexology treatment can combat a number of disorders. Tender reflexes and meridians indicate which parts of the body are congested. This assessment is of parts of the body 'out of balance', not specifically named disorders. It is important to be aware of this. Any attempt to diagnose or prescribe could well land a well-meaning reflexologist in a court of law!

Reactions to Reflexology Treatments

People differ, so do reactions – and a recipient must be informed of the possible reactions following treatment. On the whole, reactions immediately after a reflexology treatment are pleasant, leaving the patient feeling calm and relaxed or energized and rejuvenated. However, there is some bad with the good. Reflexology activates the body's own healing power, so some form of reaction is inevitable as the body rids itself of toxins. This is referred to as a 'healing crisis' and is a cleansing process. The severity of reactions depends on the degree of imbalance, but should never be too radical. The most common phrase following a first treatment is, 'I have never slept so well!'

Most common reactions are related to the body cleansing itself of toxins, so they manifest in the elimination systems of the body – the kidneys, bowels, skin and lungs. The following reactions are not unusual:

- Increased urination as the kidneys are stimulated to produce more urine, which may be darker and stronger-smelling due to the toxic content.
- Flatulence and more frequent bowel movements.
- Aggravated skin conditions, particularly in conditions which have been suppressed, such as increased perspiration and pimples.
- Improved skin tone and tissue texture due to improved circulation.
- Increased secretions of the mucous membranes in the nose, mouth and bronchioles.

- Disrupted sleep patterns – either deeper or more disturbed sleep.
- Dizziness or nausea.
- A temporary outbreak of a disease which has been suppressed.
- Increased discharge from the vagina.
- Feverishness.
- Tiredness.
- Headaches.
- Depression, overwhelming desire to weep.

Whatever the reactions, they are a necessary part of the healing process and will pass. Drinking water – preferably warm, boiled water with the juice of an organic lemon or a spoon of cider vinegar – in place of other liquids will assist in flushing toxins from the system rapidly.

Length of a Reflexology Treatment

The length of the treatment and number of sessions will vary according to the patient and the condition. The patient's constitution, history and nature of illness, age, and their body's ability to react to treatment, way of life and attitude have a profound effect on the healing process. Thus, the degree to which patients respond depends as much on themselves as on the practitioner and treatment.

The first treatment session should take approximately an hour. This is the investigative and exploratory stage, which enables you to establish as much as possible about the patient. Following treatments should last approximately 30–50 minutes, depending on the treatment required. If the session is too short, insufficient stimulus is provided for the body to mobilize its own healing powers; if it is too long, there is a danger of over-stimulation, which can cause excessive elimination and therefore discomfort.

An effect is often experienced immediately after the first treatment. Generally, results are apparent after three or four treatments – either complete or considerable improvement. Well-established disorders will take longer to eradicate than those present for a short time. A course of treatments is recommended for all conditions – even if one session appears to have corrected the problem – to balance the body totally and prevent a recurrence of the disorder. The course should be 8–12 treatments once or twice a week. For optimum results, two sessions a week are recommended until there is an improvement, and then gradually reduce the frequency. A one-off treatment will not correct problems which have been developing over several years.

If there is no reaction after several sessions, the body could be unreceptive due to external factors such as heavy medication or psychological attitude, blocking therapeutic impulses. As long as reactions are positive, there is value in continuing the treatment.

The Treatment

Once all the relevant details are noted, the treatment can proceed. As comfort is the first prerequisite, correct positioning of the therapist and patient is imperative. The patient must be seated comfortably, preferably on a soft therapy couch with the head and neck well supported, so that you are able to make eye contact. The lower legs should be well supported with the feet in a comfortable position. These should be positioned at a level comfortable for both the patient and therapist. Pillows can be used for this purpose, leaving the feet at the edge of the therapy couch with the heels hanging slightly over. In the case of children or short patients, you may have to add additional pillows behind the patient's back to move them forward. Always make sure that your patient is feeling comfortable, as they will be positioned this way for the duration of the treatment. Shoes, socks, tights and stockings must be removed and tight garments should be loosened so as not to hinder circulation.

Begin by disinfecting the feet with cotton wool soaked in disinfectant. Alternatively, use a foot spa to which a mild disinfectant has been added. Make sure the feet are completely dry prior to commencing treatment. The first physical contact is a gentle stroking movement before you proceed with a general examination of the feet. Individuals are all different, and so are their feet. Feet reveal a variety of characteristics unique to that particular patient.

Temperature, static build-up, muscle tone, tissue tone and skin condition, as well as deformities, must all be carefully noted as they all contribute to a comprehensive picture of the patient's problems. Cold, bluish or reddish feet indicate poor circulation. Sweaty feet indicate hormonal imbalance. Dry skin could indicate an imbalance with the metal element. Swelling and puffiness, especially around the ankles, can be related to a variety of internal problems. Tense feet indicate tension in the body, and limp feet indicate poor muscle tone. Foot deformities are also revealing, and are discussed in detail in a separate section of the book (see pages 226–30). Special care must be taken with broken skin conditions; these should be covered with a plaster or cotton wool before being worked on carefully. Avoid working on areas where varicose veins are present as this could further damage the veins.

Commence with a full treatment as described later in this chapter (see page 254). Working through all the reflexes activates the organs and body systems, and enables you to determine sore reflex points, which indicate areas of congestion. Eye contact is important. Most patients will react in some way – sometimes loudly – when a sore point is located. Some, however, are stubborn and refuse to react. With eye contact, you will be able to ascertain when a sensitive area is located.

The treatment must always be gentle but firm. Patients should never feel that their foot is in a vice-like grip and cannot be withdrawn. This could cause tension from a fear that treatment may be painful. There is a misunderstanding among some reflexologists that sensitive reflex points should be worked hard and brutally. This is not advisable, and the patient will probably never return. The pressure should never be more than is comfortable for the patient, but sufficiently firm to activate the body's healing potential.

Sensations vary on different parts of the feet depending on the functioning of the related body part and associated meridian/s. Congested areas will be sensitive – the more sensitive, the more congested. The sensations range from the feeling of something sharp (like a piece of glass) being pressed into the foot, to a dull ache, discomfort, tightness or just firm pressure. Sensitivity varies from person to person. For example, some people may be relatively unhealthy and have insensitive reflexes, while others may be reasonably healthy and have tender reflexes. This also varies from treatment to treatment, depending on factors such as stress, mood and time of day. In many cases, a patient may feel little or no tenderness at all during the first treatment. This does not necessarily mean that no areas are congested. More often than not, it indicates an energy blockage in the feet, which needs to be freed. The feet usually become more sensitive with subsequent treatments.

As a treatment progresses, tenderness should diminish, indicating that balance in a problem area has been restored. During treatment, you can return to reflex points already massaged if further stimulation is required. In this way, the patient is not subjected to continuous pressure on one point, which could be painful.

Only in the case of an acute pain should tight, continuous pressure be applied to the area which corresponds to the pain – for example, in cases of headache, sciatica and the like. In these instances, apply light pressure for about 15–20 seconds on the corresponding reflex. Increase the pressure until the patient is just able to tolerate the pain in the reflex area. In most cases, acute pain will disappear within a few minutes.

The Treatment Sequence

The body is reflected on the feet in a three-dimensional form. Organs overlap each other internally and therefore the same is found on the feet. Many organs are minute and not reflected on the charts, but all are worked on in the step-by-step treatment sequence. In the massage technique our school teaches, treatment always includes both feet. The reflex areas of both left and right feet are alternately massaged from toes to heel.

Many reflexologists teach the 'thumb walking' technique, and propose working one foot completely before moving on to the next. The main objective of the reflexologist is to stimulate all the reflexes on the feet. As any technique which achieves this result is equally effective, it is up to you to choose which technique works best for you. In our years of practise and teaching, we have found that the techniques illustrated here have proved their worth for both practitioner and patient. No matter what the sensations, treatment is always effective and should leave the patient feeling light, tingly and thoroughly pampered.

The most important aspect of this specific treatment procedure is that both feet are worked through alternately from top to toe. This facilitates a natural flow in the procedure. One foot represents half a body, and as many organs are paired and found on both sides of the body, it would be wrong to complete one foot at a time. This would mean that only half an organ was stimulated. The theory behind alternating feet is to stimulate each organ and body system completely before moving on to the next. In this way, each body part and system is worked as a unit even though half is on the left foot and half on the right. To execute effective reflexology massage techniques, familiarity with techniques and grips is a necessity. (Note: References to 'right' and 'left' feet mean the patient's right and left, not the therapist's.)

The detailed description of the treatment sequence that follows is included to give you a more comprehensive grasp of how to proceed easily and fluidly through the full treatment. During the treatment procedure, it is important to keep the following points in mind:

1   Always start your treatment and subsequent techniques on the right foot (unless otherwise indicated). The treatment sequence will then logically follow the mirror of the course of the colon.

2   Maintain contact with the feet at all times, especially when swapping between them.

3   Where no distinction is made as to which hand should be used as your working hand, you should make use of the hand you feel most comfortable with for that part of the sequence.

4   The support hand becomes an 'extension' of your eyes when you are unable to keep eye contact with your patient, as you will be able to feel when a patient flinches when too much pressure is exerted or when a reflex is particularly sensitive. However, be aware that this hand should not be used in lieu of regular eye contact.

5   While these techniques have been designed according to their efficacy, they can produce some form of discomfort for the patient where there are congestions. However, where a reflex is particularly sensitive, pressure should be adjusted to a level that is acceptable to the patient.

6   If for whatever reason you are unable to work on a specific area of the foot (for instance, due to severe athlete's foot or a recent broken bone), you should find a suitable referral area instead. Referral areas are those reflexes or areas that will indirectly influence the main reflex. For example, a referral area for the spine reflex will be the bladder meridian running along the lateral side of the foot.

The sitting position of therapist

Techniques have been designed not only for the benefit of the patient, but also for the therapist.

- At all times you should remain aware of your posture by keeping your spine straight and your shoulders down in a relaxed position.
- You should be able to swivel from side to side in your chair in order to work the reflexes in a comfortable manner, as not all reflexes should be worked facing the feet directly. Guidelines for the exact position of the therapist are given throughout for each step in the treatment sequence.
- Keep your feet firmly planted on the ground, with your feet spread slightly apart. Ideally, your feet should be kept in line with your shoulders, with your knees bent perpendicular.
- The feet of the patient should be resting more or less in line with your upper abdomen. If the feet are placed too high, you will not be able to keep your shoulders relaxed. Feet placed too low will cause you to bend your back, straining your muscles as a result.
- Never be scared to lean over your patient's feet and legs in order to adjust your own sitting position to a more comfortable one. Remember that constant contact with your patient is essential.

Mastering the Basics

Holding the foot

The first priority is to learn proper support or the pressure techniques will never be mastered correctly. The hands perform complementary functions throughout the treatment. While one hand presses, the other braces and supports or pushes the foot towards the pressure. The hand

applying pressure is referred to as the 'working hand', the other hand as
the 'supporting hand'. Neither hand should ever be idle.

THE STANDARD SUPPORT GRIP

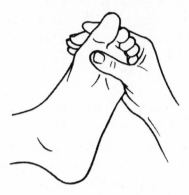

Fig. 1 The standard support grip

There is one main support technique. This is referred to as the 'standard
support grip'. Take the foot in the support hand, either from the medial or the lateral side, the web of the hand between the thumb and the
index finger touching the side of the foot, with the four fingers on the
dorsal aspect of the foot and the thumb on the plantar aspect. The support hand must always stay close to the working hand. Whichever grips
you use on whatever reflex, always keep the foot bent slightly towards
you – never in a tight grip with the toes bent backwards.

The rotating thumb technique

This is the most important technique to master, as it is used to apply
pressure to most of the reflexes throughout the treatment procedure. It
is combined with finger techniques.

Before working on the feet, try the 'rotating thumb technique' on the
palm of your hand. It helps to visualize the object being worked on

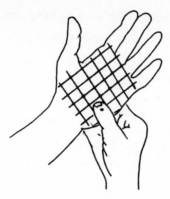

Fig. 2 Rotating thumb technique

(hand or foot) divided into small squares, all of which must be systematically stimulated. As you work, move from square to square, applying pressure and rotation to each square. The movement of the thumb from point to point must be small, moving along progressively, leaving no space between the points covered by the thumb tip.

For this exercise, place the four fingers of the working hand on the dorsal aspect of the hand to be worked on, keeping the thumb free to work on the palm. Bend the thumb from the first joint to a 75–90° angle – the angle must ensure that the thumbnail does not dig into the flesh. This is the standard position of the rotating thumb. The contact point is the tip of the thumb. Apply firm pressure with the tip of the thumb to the point to be worked on, and rotate the thumb, clockwise or anti-clockwise. Keep the pressure firm and constant and stay on the square. Two to three rotations are sufficient. Lift the thumb, move to the next point and repeat the procedure. The basic movement is: press in, rotate, lift, move. The amount of pressure and number of rotations depend on the patient's foot size.

Observe the movement of the thumb on the working hand. The most visible rotation must be at the second thumb joint – where the metacarpals of the hand join the phalanges of the thumb. Two basic tenets for ease in executing this technique are to keep the thumb bent and the shoulders down. There should be very little strain on the arm muscles, elbows, neck and shoulders.

Furthermore, you will notice how much more pressure can be applied with the thumb in a bent position as opposed to a flat thumb. By exercising the correct technique, the treatment procedure should not be at all strenuous for the practitioner. Practise this thumb rotating technique on your hand until you feel completely comfortable with it. Also ensure that you exercise the thumbs on both hands to enable you to work efficiently with either thumb, as it is important to be able to switch hands during the treatment sequence.

Relaxation

The first step in the treatment procedure is to relax the patient, release tension from the ankles and loosen the feet. Alternating feet for each technique, sitting in a position where you are facing the feet of the patient directly, begin with the relaxation techniques in the following order:

1. ACHILLES TENDON STRETCH

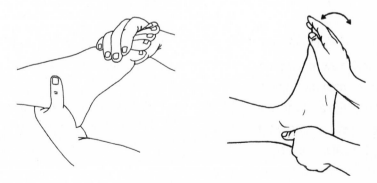

Fig. 3 Achilles tendon stretch

Cup the heel of one foot so that it rests in the palm of the supporting hand. Grasp the top of the foot near the toes in the standard support grip. Pull the foot towards you, allowing the heel to move backwards, and then reverse the procedure, pulling the heel towards you and pushing the foot backwards by placing the palm of the working hand against the plantar aspect of the foot, so that the Achilles tendon at the back of the heel stretches out. Repeat this technique two or three times on each foot.

Therapist position: Face the feet directly, with your arms kept loosely at your sides. Keep your shoulders relaxed, your spine straight and your elbows down. Your feet should be placed squarely on the ground, slightly apart. Remember to keep intermittent eye contact with your patient (see page 255).

2. ANKLE ROTATION

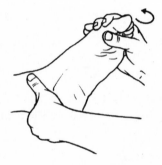

Fig. 4 Ankle rotation

Cup the heel and the posterior aspect of the ankle of the foot to be worked on in the palm of the support hand, with the fingers on one side of the foot and the thumb on the other. Ensure you use a firm but not tight grasp. The working hand grasps the foot at the base of the toes in the standard support grip. Hold the foot with equal pressure. Use the support hand as a pivot and rotate the foot with the working hand in 360° circles, clockwise and anticlockwise a few times. Work the other foot the same way.

Do not force the foot into exaggerated circles; manoeuvre it slowly and gently as far as is comfortable for the patient. It affects the entire area of the hip joint, tailbone and surrounding areas, as well as all the lower back muscles.

Therapist position: Face the feet directly, with your arms kept loosely at your sides. Keep your shoulders relaxed, your spine straight and your elbows down. Your feet should be placed squarely on the ground, slightly apart. Remember to keep eye contact with your patient.

3. SIDE TO SIDE

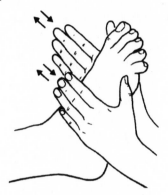

Fig. 5 Side to side

Place your palms on either side of the foot close to the toes. Keep the hands as relaxed and loose as possible. Roll the foot from side to side by gently moving it back and forth between your palms, which move in opposite directions from each other. The sole of the foot should 'clap' against the palm of the hands when performing this technique. Do not force the foot to roll farther than is comfortable for the patient. Move the hands gradually down the sides of the foot until the entire foot is worked. This is usually executed vigorously to release tension, relax the edges of the ankle and calf, and stimulate the whole foot.

Therapist position: Face the feet directly, with your arms kept loosely at your sides. Keep your shoulders relaxed, your spine straight and your elbows down. Your feet should be placed squarely on the ground, slightly apart. Remember to keep eye contact with your patient.

4. LOOSEN ANKLES

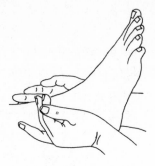

Fig. 6 Loosen ankles

Lock the sides of both palms below the anklebones, covering these with the palms of your hands. The fingers are placed loosely against the lower leg. The ankle joint serves as the pivot point. Move the hands rapidly backwards and forwards in opposite directions to each other, keeping the hands locked beneath the anklebones. Note: The foot will shake from side to side when this movement is properly executed.

Therapist position: Face the feet directly, with your arms kept loosely at your sides. Keep your shoulders relaxed, your spine straight and your elbows down. Your feet should be placed squarely on the ground, slightly apart. Remember to keep eye contact with your patient.

5. WRINGING THE FOOT

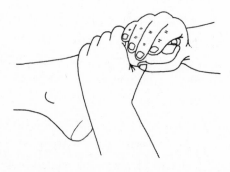

Fig. 7 Wringing the foot

Clasp the foot from opposite directions in both hands as you would a wet towel and wring gently, each hand twisting in opposite directions. Be careful not to pull the skin when performing this technique – the object is to open up the area between the bones of the foot. The thumbs push the foot upwards, allowing the foot to be bent down at the medial and lateral sides. Move the hands gradually up or down the foot to 'wring' the entire foot.

Therapist position: Face the feet directly, with your arms kept loosely at your sides. Keep your shoulders relaxed and your spine straight. Your elbows should fly up and down when you perform this technique. Your feet should be placed squarely on the ground, slightly apart. Remember to keep eye contact with your patient.

6. ROTATE ALL TOES

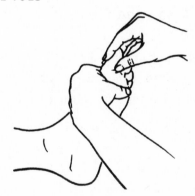

Fig. 8 Rotate all toes

This relaxation technique not only increases flexibility of the toes, but also releases tension and loosens muscles in the neck and shoulder line. The big toe is the most important here as it represents the neck area.

To execute this procedure, begin with the big toe and work through all the toes of one foot before moving on to the other foot. Hold the foot with the support hand in the standard support grip. The four fingers of the working hand are placed on the dorsal aspect of the toes, with the thumb grasping the base of the toe from below at the phalange joint. Now gently pull the toe in its joint with a slight upward movement, pulling the foot at the same time downward with the support hand, as if you were separating the toe from the foot. Rotate in 360° circles, clockwise or anticlockwise a few times. Rotations must be gentle but firm, the support hand stabilizing the toes at the metatarsals.

Therapist position: Face the feet directly, with your arms kept loosely at your sides. Keep your shoulders relaxed and your spine straight. The elbow of your working hand will lift up approximately to shoulder level, with the elbow of the support hand being kept down. Your feet should be placed squarely on the ground, slightly apart. Remember to keep eye contact with your patient.

Head and Neck Area – the Toes and their Meridians

The toes represent the head and neck area. Reflexes found here include the sinuses, pituitary gland, brain matter (which also includes the reflexes for the pineal gland and hypothalamus), neck, eyes and ears.

Sinuses

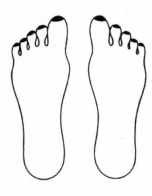
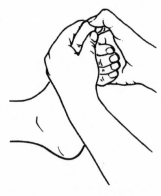

Fig. 9a Sinuses   *Fig. 9b Grip A*

GRIP A

Place the dorsal side of the four fingers of your working hand against the ball of the foot to be worked on and bend them loosely at the second joint. The thumb is now free to work on the tips of the toes in the rotating thumb position. The fingers of the working hand will provide additional support on the ball of the foot. The rotating thumb technique is used to exert pressure on the reflex points. The support hand is in the standard support position close to the working hand. However, hold each toe individually at the base of the toe (phalangeal joint) with the support hand as you work them, to prevent the toes from moving and bending. With Grip A, the left hand is usually the support hand and the right hand the worker.

The sinus reflexes are situated on the tips of the toes. Work these from the big to the small toe, first on the right foot, then the left. Starting on the big toe, apply the thumb rotation technique – press in, rotate, lift and move. The area to cover on each toe is the equivalent of three to five small 'squares', depending on the size of the toe. The support hand moves along with the working hand, at the same time leaving enough space for the working hand to work in effectively and provide additional support against the ball of the foot.

Therapist position: Face the feet directly, with your arms kept loosely at your sides. Keep your shoulders relaxed, your spine straight and your elbows down. Your feet should be placed squarely on the ground, slightly apart. Remember to keep eye contact with your patient.

Pituitary gland

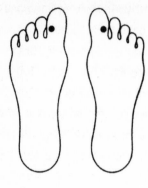

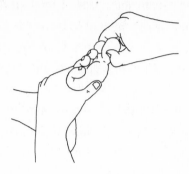

Fig. 10a Pituitary gland   Fig. 10b Grip B

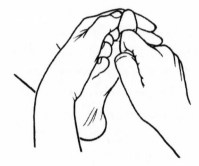

Fig. 10c Grip C

GRIP B

Here the support hand holds the foot in the standard support grip close to the toes. With the working hand, place the palmar aspect of the fingers on the dorsal aspect of the foot pointing towards the ankle. The thumb is then free to work on the reflex of the pituitary gland embedded in the cushion of the big toe with the rotating thumb technique.

GRIP C

This is an alternative grip with which to locate and stimulate the pituitary gland if you have trouble with Grip B. Bend the index finger at the second joint and use this as you would the thumb. The support hand cups the toes from the dorsal side, pushing the foot towards the pressure. Find the reflex, press in, rotate clockwise or anticlockwise a few times, and then release pressure when you feel the reflex has been sufficiently stimulated.

The pituitary gland reflex is situated within the brain reflex on the big toe. The exact point must be located and individually worked on to stimulate the endocrine system. (see section on Mapping, page 189 on how to locate this point) Sometimes this reflex is clearly visible as a small mound. A sharp pain marks the site of this reflex, so there will be no mistaking it.

Therapist position: Face the feet directly, with your arms kept loosely at your sides. Keep your shoulders relaxed and your spine straight. The elbow of your working hand will lift up approximately to shoulder level, with the elbow of the support hand being kept down. Your feet should be placed squarely on the ground, slightly apart. Remember to keep eye contact with your patient. Note: When using grip C, keep your arms loosely at your sides. Keep your shoulders relaxed, your spine straightened and your elbows down.

Brain matter, neck, eyes and ears

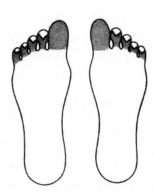

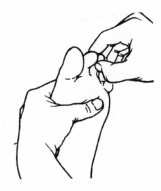

Fig. 11a Brain matter, neck, eyes and ears

Fig. 11b Grip B

GRIP B

The support hand holds the foot in the standard support grip close to the toes. With the working hand, place the palmar aspect of the fingers on the dorsal aspect of the foot pointing towards the ankle. The thumb is then free to work on the reflexes on the cushions of all the toes with the rotating thumb technique.

Return to the big toe of the right foot, and work the brain matter and neck reflexes areas with Grip B. Cover the entire area to the base of the big toe using this technique, right down to where the ball of the foot starts. Then proceed to work on the eye and ear reflexes on the four toes of the same foot, before moving to the other foot to repeat the procedure.

The eye reflexes are situated around the cushions of the second and third toes; the ear reflexes around the cushions of the fourth and fifth toes. Imagine the cushions of the toes as inverted triangles. The thumb must work on the three points of the triangles, which are situated almost 'under' the cushions. First, work the medial point, then the middle followed by the lateral point. Without breaking the flow, continue with the rotating thumb down the shaft of the toe to the base of the metatarsal/phalange joint. Complete this procedure on each toe before moving to the next one. You will often find an undue amount of pain in this area. This may not necessarily relate to imbalances in the eyes or ears, but to congestion along the meridian related to each of the toes. Always support around the base of the toes as they are worked on to prevent them from bending.

Therapist position: Face the feet directly, keeping your shoulders relaxed and spine straight. The elbow of your working hand will gradually lift approximately to shoulder level as you work the triangles around the cushions of the second to fourth toes, with the elbow of the support hand remaining down. Your feet should be placed squarely on the ground, slightly apart. Remember to keep eye contact with your patient.

Sides and dorsal aspects of toes – the meridians

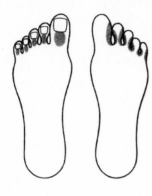

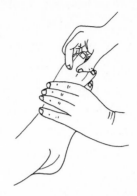

Fig. 12a Sides and dorsal
aspects of toes

Fig. 12b Finger technique 1

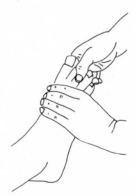

Fig. 12c Grip D

FINGER TECHNIQUE 1

This technique is used on the sides of the toes. Pull the foot down towards you with the support hand in the standard support position close to the toes, far enough so that the toes are almost in a horizontal position as opposed to being vertical. However, if the patient's foot is relatively immobile or bending the foot becomes painful, you should change to a standing position. Place the pad of the index finger on one side and the pad of the thumb on the other side at the base of the toe to be worked on. Squeeze and rotate both the index finger and thumb simultaneously on either side of the toe, rotating in the same direction. Rotate, lift and move up to the tip of the toes.

GRIP D

Pull the foot down towards you with the support hand in the standard support position close to the toes, far enough so that the toes are almost in a horizontal position as opposed to being vertical. With the working hand, place the palmar aspect of the fingers against the ball of the foot pointing towards the ankle. The thumb is then free to work on the meridians on the dorsal aspect of all the toes with the rotating thumb technique, starting at the base of each toe.

Imagine the toes as being square in shape. Ensure that the sides of each toe are worked thoroughly from the base to the tip of the toes, starting from the big toe and ending with the little toe. The dorsal side of the toes is stimulated with Grip D on the same foot, from the big toe to the little toe. Repeat the full procedure on the left foot. It is important to massage the toes thoroughly, as this will stimulate the six main meridians thoroughly.

Therapist position: Face the feet directly, with your arms kept loosely at your sides. Keep your shoulders relaxed, your spine straight and your elbows down. Your feet should be placed squarely on the ground, slightly apart. Remember to keep eye contact with your patient. If the patient's feet are rigid, still or painful, change to a standing position, keeping your feet spread slightly apart.

Eustachian tube, chronic eyes and ears

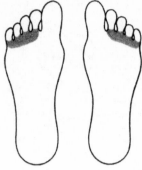

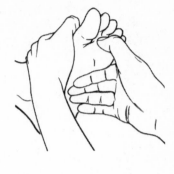

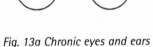

Fig. 13a Chronic eyes and ears

Fig. 13b Grip A

GRIP A

Place the dorsal side of the four fingers of your working hand against the arch of the foot to be worked on and bend them loosely at the second joint. The thumb is now free to work at the base of the toes in the rotating thumb position. The fingers of the working hand will provide additional support in the arch of the foot. The rotating thumb technique is used to exert pressure on the reflex points. The support hand cups the foot from the dorsal side, pushing the foot towards the pressure. With Grip A, the left hand is usually the support hand and the right hand the worker.

If you bend the foot fractionally forward with the support hand, a distinct 'shelf' will be visible at the base of the toes. This is the section to be worked on. With the rotating thumb technique move from point to point along the shelf from the web of the big toe to the fifth toe. Repeat this procedure on both feet.

Therapist position: Face the feet directly, with your arms kept loosely at your sides. Keep your shoulders relaxed, your spine straight and your elbows down. Your feet should be placed squarely on the ground, slightly apart. Remember to keep eye contact with your patient.

Upper lymphatic system

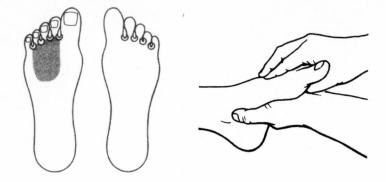

Fig. 14a Upper lymphatic system   Fig. 14b Finger technique 2

FINGER TECHNIQUE 2

Cup the arch of the foot in the palm of the support hand, pulling the foot down towards you until the toes are in a more horizontal position. Place the middle finger on top of the index finger to enable you to exert greater pressure on the lymphatic system reflexes. The pad of the index finger is responsible for the rotations on the dorsal aspect of the foot. Move the working hand in between the toes, positioning the web between the index finger and thumb against the web between the toes. The thumb of the working hand provides extra support on the plantar aspect of the foot.

Reach as far down the foot as possible with the working fingers and, using the rotation movement as you would with the thumb, work point by point towards the webs. When you reach the webs, apply a tight, pinching and rotating pressure on the webs as these are important lymphatic drainage points. Repeat this between each toe, using the grooves between the metatarsal bones as guidelines. The support hand should follow the working hand as it moves along.

The most important lymphatic system reflexes are located in the webs between the toes, but the entire area on the dorsal aspect of the foot –

from the ankle joint to the webs – must be worked on for optimum stimulation. This will work many important acupuncture points located on the meridians at the same time. When working between the big and second toes, work down the side of the big toe up to the phalange-metatarsal joint to stimulate the tonsil reflexes as well.

Many people suffer from congestion in the lymphatic system and the meridians found in these areas, and will usually be sensitive in these places. The reflex between the dorsal aspect of the big and second toes is also the oesophagus reflex area and will be particularly sensitive on smokers.

Therapist position: Face the feet directly. Remember to pull the patient's foot downwards towards you with the support hand, so that you do not work the reflexes at an awkward angle. Keep your shoulders relaxed, your spine straight and your elbows down. Your feet should be placed squarely on the ground, slightly apart. Remember to keep eye contact with your patient.

Thoracic Area – the Ball

The thoracic area covers the balls of both feet and extends from the base of the toes to the end of the ball. The division between the ball and the arch is clearly demarcated and corresponds to the diaphragm reflex. In the body, the diaphragm separates the thoracic cavity from the abdominal cavity.

Reflexes situated here: lungs, heart, shoulders, bronchi, thyroid, parathyroid, oesophagus (including trachea and thymus) and diaphragm.

Bronchi, lungs and heart

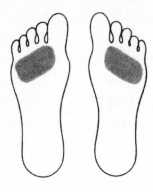

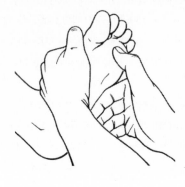

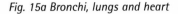

Fig. 15a Bronchi, lungs and heart   Fig. 15b Grip A

GRIP A

Place the dorsal side of the four fingers of your working hand against the arch of the foot to be worked on and bend them loosely at the second joint. The thumb is now free to work on the ball of the foot in the rotating thumb position. The fingers of the working hand will provide additional support in the arch of the foot. The rotating thumb technique is used to exert pressure on the reflex points. The support hand cups the foot from the dorsal side, pushing the foot towards the pressure. You can use either hand as the working hand, swapping between them where necessary to work the reflexes.

The bronchi and lung reflexes are situated on the ball of both feet, extending from below the second toe to just beyond the fourth toe. The heart is a single organ found on the left side of the body, therefore the heart reflex is found on the left foot only. As the thyroid reflex covers a large part of the ball of the foot (see page 275), this reflex will also be partially stimulated when working the section underneath the big toe.

Start working on the ball just below the neck area of the big toe on the right foot. You can move from right to left and back again, or up and down this area, as long as the entire ball of the foot is covered, including the shoulder and thyroid reflex areas. The heart reflex is lodged in the lung reflex area of the left foot, just above the diaphragm line to the lateral aspect of the solar plexus reflex, which is also found on the internal kidney meridian (see page 197).

Therapist position: Face the feet directly, with your arms kept loosely at your sides. Keep your shoulders relaxed, your spine straight and your elbows down. Your feet should be placed squarely on the ground, slightly apart. Remember to keep eye contact with your patient.

Thyroid, parathyroid and oesophagus

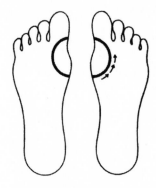
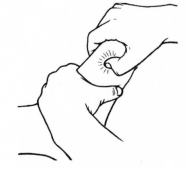

Fig. 16a Thyroid, parathyroid and oesophagus

Fig. 16b Grip E

GRIP E

Grasp the foot with both hands from the instep of the foot – fingers on the dorsal aspect, thumbs on the plantar aspect. The hand closest to the ankle is used as the support hand in the standard support grip. The fingers of the working hand bend the foot slightly forward, while the thumb is kept free to work 'up and under' the bone of the metatarsal-phalange joint using the rotating thumb technique.

The thyroid reflex covers the entire area of the ball of the foot below the big toe, but the most important part is found in the half-circle shape at the base of the ball, almost under the bone of the metatarsal-phalange joint. The reflex area is covered in a circular movement – starting from the medial aspect of the foot. To achieve sufficient stimulation, you must get right into the bone and press 'up and under'. Continue up to the base of the big toe along the oesophagus reflex. Move across and then down to work the parathyroid reflex, before moving back to the starting point to complete the circle. The main or primary thyroid reflex, situated specifically round the base of the ball of the foot is often sensitive, so proceed with care.

Therapist position: Swivel in your chair so as to face the feet at an angle from the medial side. Keep your shoulders relaxed and your spine straight. The elbow of the working hand moves out and up to above shoulder level to facilitate the angle necessary to get right into the thyroid reflex. Your feet should be placed squarely on the ground, slightly apart. Remember to keep eye contact with your patient.

The diaphragm

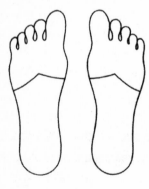

Fig. 17a The diaphragm

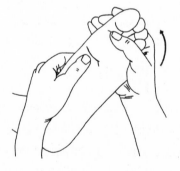

Fig. 17b Grip F

GRIP F

With the support hand in the standard support grip, grasp the top of the foot from the lateral side. The working hand grasps the foot from the instep, placing the four fingers on the dorsal side of the foot. The thumb is kept slightly bent and the tip of the thumb is placed on the diaphragm reflex. The thumb pushes under the metatarsal bone at a slight angle while the support hand lifts and pulls the foot towards you in an 'up and over', wave-like manner.

The diaphragm separates the thoracic cavity from the abdominal cavity in the body. Its corresponding reflex separates the ball of the foot from the arch. Start on the medial aspect of the foot in line with the big toe, using the thumb and lifting action and proceed along the diaphragm line. The thumb will automatically work up and under the metatarsal bones at a slight angle.

Therapist position: Face the feet directly, keeping your shoulders relaxed and your spine straight. The elbow of the working hand moves out and up to just below shoulder level to facilitate the lifting movement. Your feet should be placed squarely on the ground, slightly apart. Remember to keep eye contact with your patient.

The Abdominal Area – the Arch

All the reflexes related to the digestive system are located in the arch of the foot. This section is often very sensitive to pressure. Reflexes here are:

Above the waistline: Right foot – liver, gall bladder, stomach, pancreas, duodenum, kidney, adrenal gland. Left foot – stomach, pancreas, duodenum, spleen, kidney, adrenal gland.

Below the waistline: Right foot – appendix, ileo-caecal valve, ascending colon, transverse colon, small intestine, ureter, bladder. Left foot – transverse colon, descending colon, sigmoid flexure, rectum, anus, small intestine, ureter, bladder.

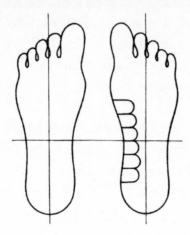

Fig. 18 Dividing the arch of the foot

As this is a rather complex area, with organs close to and overlapping each other, I have devised a method that I find simplifies locating the organ reflexes.

The arch is clearly visible on the plantar aspect of the foot – the raised area, which extends from the base of the ball to the beginning of the heel. This section of the foot is roughly the equivalent of six thumb widths (of the patient's thumb) measured horizontally. If the practitioner's thumb is approximately the same size as the patient's, the divisions will be perfectly accurate. The first three thumb widths on the inside of the foot cover the reflexes of the stomach, pancreas and duodenum respectively. These end at the waistline. The three measures below the waistline cover the large and small intestine.

Liver and gall bladder

GRIP G

For the liver and gall bladder reflexes, the right supporting hand will hold the foot in the standard support grip close to the toes. The left

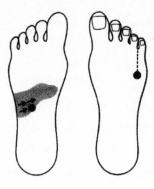 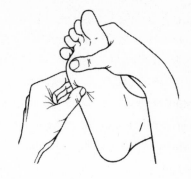

Fig. 19a Liver and gall bladder   *Fig. 19b Grip G*

working hand grasps the foot from the lateral side, with the four fingers on the dorsal side and the thumb positioned to work the liver and gall bladder reflexes. This grip requires the thumb to work the reflexes on the foot at a horizontal angle. The pressure is, as usual, exerted with the rotating thumb technique.

The liver is the largest organ inside the body, thus the reflex covers a large area. It is situated on the right foot only. The gall bladder reflex is close to and often embedded in the liver reflex – it is so close as to be almost indistinguishable. To locate the liver reflex, imagine a triangle below the ball of the foot. One side of the triangle lies at the lateral edge of the foot, the other at the diaphragm line. The base of the triangle cuts diagonally across the arch. This line merges the liver reflex into those of the stomach, pancreas and duodenum.

The gall bladder reflex is more difficult to locate. Reference to the section on meridians will help clarify this location (see page 152). Run your index finger up towards the ankle between the fourth and fifth toes. In the web between the metatarsals, you will find a slight indentation, which will be particularly sensitive to pressure. This is an acupuncture point on the gall bladder meridian. Once this is located, pinpoint the area directly beneath on the plantar aspect of the foot with your thumb

– this is the gall bladder reflex. In some people this is in the middle of the liver reflex. This exercise is not necessary every time you give a treatment. Use it to differentiate the gall bladder reflex from the liver reflex if there is sensitivity in this area.

Start working from the lateral side of the foot and work towards the midline. You can move from left to right and back again, or up and down this area, as long as the entire lateral half of the arch above the waistline of the foot is covered, including the overlapping stomach, pancreas and duodenum reflexes.

Therapist position: To execute this grip effectively, you must be seated in such a way as to be able to swivel in your seat and face the foot to be worked on at an angle from the medial side. The arm of the right support hand rests across the patient's left leg. Your shoulders should be kept relaxed, your spine straight and the elbow of your working hand slightly elevated. Your feet should be placed squarely on the ground, slightly apart. Remember to keep eye contact with your patient.

Stomach, pancreas, duodenum, spleen

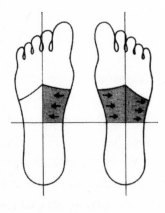

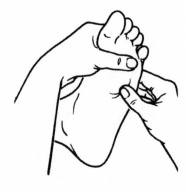

*Fig. 20a Stomach, pancreas,
duodenum and spleen*

Fig. 20b Grip G

GRIP G

When utilizing Grip G, always work the outside of the foot with the 'outer' hand and support with the 'inner' hand from the instep, and vice versa. The working hand grasps the foot from the medial side, with the four fingers on the dorsal side and the thumb positioned to work the stomach, pancreas and duodenum reflexes. This grip requires the thumb to start working the foot at a more horizontal angle. The pressure is, as usual, exerted with the rotating thumb.

The stomach, pancreas and duodenum reflexes are found on both feet. The spleen reflex is on the left foot only opposite to the liver reflex, but is a lot smaller and more in line with the stomach and pancreas reflexes. To locate the reflexes use the thumb measure rule (the patient's thumb) – the first thumb width nearest the ball of the foot pinpoints the stomach, the second the pancreas, and the third the duodenum reflex, ending directly above the waistline.

On the right foot, use your left hand in the standard support grip. The thumb of the right hand starts working from the medial aspect of the foot and moves inward to the midline, working through the stomach reflex. Repeat this procedure for the pancreas and duodenum reflexes. As only a small portion of these three reflexes are found on the right foot, complete the right foot first before moving over to the left foot.

Now the right hand is the 'outside' support hand and the left hand works the medial aspect of the foot across the stomach reflex to the halfway mark or imaginary vertical midline. At this point, swap hands to work the lateral aspect of the foot on the same thumb width to work the remainder of the stomach reflex as well as part of the spleen reflex. Repeat the same action to work the pancreas and duodenum reflexes. The relatively small spleen reflex will be stimulated at the same time, as will a small portion of the large intestine reflex.

Therapist position: To execute this grip effectively, you must be seated in such a way as to be able to swivel in your seat and face the foot to be worked on at an angle from the medial side. Start off with the arm of the right working hand resting across the patient's left leg. Your shoulders should be kept relaxed, your spine straight and the elbow of your support hand kept loosely at your side. Your feet should be placed squarely on the ground, slightly apart. When moving over to the left foot, swivel round in your chair to face the feet from the medial aspect, resting your left arm across the patient's right leg. The right elbow is kept loosely at your side or slightly elevated, depending on which hand is used as the working hand. Remember to keep eye contact with your patient.

Small intestine, ileo-caecal valve, appendix, large intestine, rectum and anus

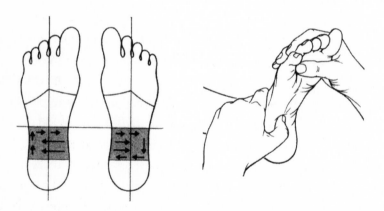

Fig. 21a Small intestine, ileo-caecal valve, appendix, large intestine, rectum and anus

Fig. 21b Grip G

GRIP G

When utilizing Grip G, always work the outside of the foot with the 'outer' hand and support with the 'inner' hand from the instep, and vice versa. The working hand grasps the foot with the four fingers on the dorsal side and the thumb positioned to work the small intestine, ileo-caecal valve, appendix, large intestine, and rectum and anus reflexes. This grip requires the thumb to start working the foot at a more horizontal angle. The pressure is, as usual, exerted with the rotating thumb.

The small and large intestine reflexes are found on both feet. The ileo-caecal valve and appendix reflexes are found on the right foot only, with the rectum and anus reflex being on the left foot. To locate the reflexes use the thumb measure rule – the fourth thumb width, positioned underneath the waistline, relates to the transverse colon, with the fifth and sixth thumb widths relating to the small intestine on both feet. The ascending and descending colon are found on the lateral aspect of the right and left foot respectively, in line with the fifth and sixth thumb widths.

The small intestine joins the large intestine at the ileo-caecal valve below the fourth toe in the sixth thumb width. This valve plays an important part in digestion. If it is not functioning properly, food particles can enter the large intestine before all the nutrients have been absorbed, or particles from the large intestine may filter back into the small intestine, which could cause infection of the appendix. The appendix reflex is slightly below the ileo-caecal valve reflex.

On the left foot, use your right hand in the standard support grip. Start working the small intestine reflex on the medial aspect of the left foot on the fifth thumb width position, supporting with the left hand and working the instep with the right hand. Work the entire 'square' towards the lateral aspect of the foot, until you reach one thumb width away from the lateral edge. Keep the thumb in a horizontal position and work two to three horizontal rows. There is no need to change hands at the midline as the working thumb should be able to stretch far enough across to cover the entire reflex. When work on the small intestine area is completed on the left foot, repeat the procedure on the right foot. You will need to swap around the working and supporting hands in order to do so.

The reflexes for the large intestine are worked on in the same directions as it functions in the body – up the ascending, across the transverse and down the descending colon to the rectum. Because food particles can easily become lodged in the corners (flexures), these areas must be worked on firmly to stimulate the flow.

Still using Grip G, start on the right foot at the heel line just below the ileo-caecal valve/appendix reflex. Remember to keep your thumb in a horizontal position throughout when working these reflexes. The left hand works on the lateral aspect of the foot, while the right hand supports from the medial side in the standard support grip with the arm resting across the patient's left leg. Work the rotating thumb up to the liver reflex (hepatic flexure) in the fourth thumb width, then work across to cover the transverse colon. Work with the left hand to the imaginary vertical midline, then change to work with the right hand and support with the left hand.

The transverse colon continues on the left foot. The left arm is now resting across the patient's right leg. Support with the 'outside' right hand and work with the 'inside' left hand, until you reach the midline of the foot. Then change hands again and work with the 'outside' right hand and support with the 'inside' left hand to complete the transverse colon reflex area. Continue down from below the spleen reflex (splenic flexure) to work the descending colon on the lateral side of the foot. The reflex curves into the sigmoid flexure and continues to the rectum/anus reflex. Change working hands whenever necessary for your own comfort when reaching this point. Once this section is complete, the entire digestive system has been stimulated.

Therapist position: To execute this grip effectively, you must be seated in such a way as to be able to swivel in your seat and face the foot to be worked on at an angle from the medial side. Start off with the arm of the left working hand resting across the patient's right leg. Your shoulders should be kept relaxed, your spine straight and the elbow of your support hand kept loosely at your side. When using your right hand as the working hand for the large intestine reflex, the elbow will be slightly elevated. Your feet should be placed squarely on the ground, slightly apart. When moving over to the right foot, swivel round in your chair to once again face the feet from the medial aspect, resting your right arm across the patient's left leg. The left elbow is kept loosely at your side or slightly elevated, depending on which hand is used as the working hand. Remember to keep eye contact with your patient.

Kidneys, adrenal glands and ureters

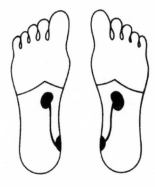 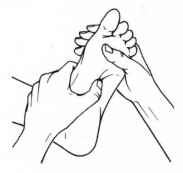

Fig. 22a Kidneys, adrenal glands
and ureters

Fig. 22b Grip G

GRIP G

The 'inner' working hand grasps the foot with the four fingers on the dorsal side and the thumb positioned to work the kidney and ureter reflexes. This grip requires the thumb to start working the foot at a more horizontal angle. The pressure is, as usual, exerted with the rotating thumb. The support hand is held in the standard support grip near the toes.

Bladder

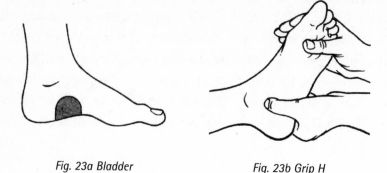

Fig. 23a Bladder

Fig. 23b Grip H

GRIP H

The support hand remains in the standard support grip. Cup the instep towards the heel of the foot in the palm of the working hand, pulling the foot down towards you with the support hand until the toes are in a more horizontal position. The thumb is left free on the medial aspect of the foot to execute the rotating thumb technique, with the four fingers supporting the foot on the lateral side.

The kidneys are paired organs, so reflexes are found on both feet. The adrenal gland reflexes are directly above the kidney reflexes so they are worked simultaneously with the kidneys. To locate the kidney reflex, first find the solar plexus reflex. This is in the central indentation on the diaphragm line of the ball of the foot. The kidney reflex is approximately one thumb measure below this.

The ureter reflex is often mapped on the foot with small grooves in the skin as a curved line descending across the arch towards the bladder reflex under the medial anklebone. The bladder reflex is roughly the size of a large coin and is often puffy, particularly if there is a bladder imbalance.

Even though the kidney reflex is situated below the solar plexus, start working from the solar plexus reflex, as it is the first acupuncture point along the actual kidney meridian. This meridian descends down the arch of the foot along the ureter and through the bladder reflex, so it would make sense to start at this point. Position your thumb on the solar plexus, rotate, lift and move down further to the kidney and adrenal glands, then along the ureter tube towards the bladder at the edge of the heel. Work this area with Grip G until you reach the bladder reflex, then change to Grip H. This changeover is made in a single movement so as not to break the flow of the treatment. Repeat the same procedure on the left foot.

Therapist position: To execute this grip effectively, you must be seated in such a way as to be able to swivel in your seat and face the foot to be worked on at an angle from the medial side. The arm of the working hand rests across the patient's leg. Your shoulders should be kept relaxed, your spine straight and the elbow of your support hand loosely at your sides. Your feet should be placed squarely on the ground, slightly apart. When changing to Grip H, change your seating position at the same time to face the feet directly. The arms of the support and working hands will no longer use the legs of the patient as a 'resting tool' – they are kept loosely at your sides with your elbows down. Remember to keep eye contact with your patient.

The Pelvic Area – the Heel

The pelvic area is the toughest to work on, as the skin is often hard due to the fact that the heel bears the brunt of the body weight when walking. As a result, few people feel any sensation in this area. This does not detract from the fact that it is important to work this area well. Many suffer from congestions here and these may be aggravated by the presence of numerous meridians in the pelvic area of the body. These meridians penetrate all of the organs positioned in the pelvic cavity of the body. It is a frequent occurrence for organs in the body to become prolapsed to some extent, causing, for example, some digestive organs to move down in the pelvic cavity – hence the importance to stimulate the entire heel thoroughly.

Pelvis and sciatic nerve

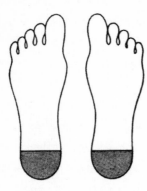

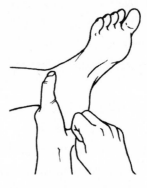

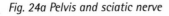

Fig. 24a Pelvis and sciatic nerve   Fig. 24b Knead technique

KNEAD TECHNIQUE

This is a relatively easy technique to master. It is used mainly on the heel area, which is usually rather tough, and therefore needs more pressure for effective stimulation. Cup the ankle in the palm of the support hand, keeping the heel area free. Make a loose fist with the working hand, and then use the second joint of the index and/or middle fingers to 'knead' the heels as you would dough.

The sciatic reflex and nerve run horizontally across the heel so it will be stimulated automatically as the heel is worked on. If the patient has very soft heels, you can use the rotating thumb technique instead.

Therapist position: Face the feet directly, with your arms kept loosely at your sides. Keep your shoulders relaxed, your spine straight and your elbows down. Your feet should be placed squarely on the ground, slightly apart. Remember to keep eye contact with your patient.

Reproductive Area – the Ankles

All the reproductive organ reflexes are situated around the ankle area (see pages 206–9). The kidney and bladder meridians also penetrate the ankle area. The reflexes found here are: ovaries, uterus and Fallopian tubes (females) and testes, prostate and vas deferens (males).

Uterus/prostate and ovaries/testes

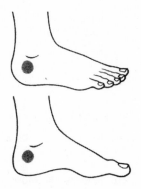

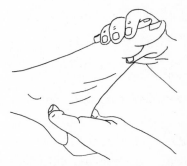

Fig. 25a Ovaries/testes and
uterus/prostate

Fig. 25b Grip H

GRIP H

The support hand is held in the standard support grip. Cup the instep towards the heel of the foot in the palm of the working hand, pulling the foot down towards you with the support hand until the toes are in a more horizontal position. The thumb is left free to execute the rotating thumb technique, with the four fingers supporting on the opposite side of the foot.

Fallopian tubes/vas deferens and lymphatic system (groin area)

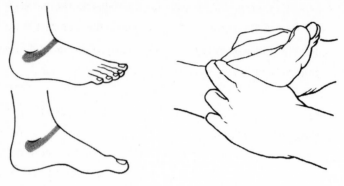

*Fig. 26a Fallopian tubes/vas deferens
and lymphatic system (groin area)*

Fig. 26b Finger technique 3

FINGER TECHNIQUE 3

The hands are placed on opposite sides of the foot with the thumbs on the plantar aspect and the four fingers of each hand on the dorsal aspect. The index and middle fingers are the working tools. The middle finger is placed on top of the index finger to create extra leverage. With the fingers, press in, rotate, lift and move, point by point as with the rotating thumb technique.

The uterus and prostate reflexes are located on the medial aspect of the foot below the anklebone. To find the position of this reflex, find the medial aspect on the posterior side of the heel. Connect this point with the anklebone in a diagonal line – the reflex is situated in the hollow area between these two points. The ovaries/testes reflex can be found in the same way on the lateral aspect of the foot.

The Fallopian tubes/vas deferens and lymphatic system reflexes run from just below the lateral ankle bone, across the superior aspect of the foot to beneath the medial ankle bone, linking the reproductive organs with one another. The lymphatic system reflexes found in the groin area are found in the same band across the foot, just above the Fallopian tube/vas deferens reflexes.

To work this area, use Grip H as with the bladder. The supporting right hand pulls the foot down in the standard support grip, with the left hand cupping the instep to work the uterus reflex on the medial aspect of the foot. The area to cover is approximately the size of a large coin. Change hands to work the ovaries/testes reflex on the lateral aspect of the same foot.

The Fallopian tube/vas deferens reflexes are then worked with both hands using Finger Technique 3, starting from just below the ankle bones in the uterus/prostate and ovaries/testes reflexes and meeting at the superior aspect of the foot. The lymphatic system reflexes found in the groin area will be stimulated at the same time. Repeat the whole procedure on the left foot.

Therapist position: Face the feet directly, with your arms kept loosely at your sides. Keep your shoulders relaxed, your spine straight and your elbows down. Your feet should be placed squarely on the ground, slightly apart. Remember to keep eye contact with your patient.

The Spine – Medial Foot

The spinal twist

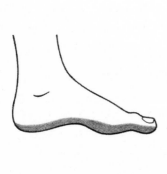

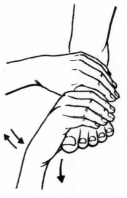

Fig. 27a Spine

Fig. 27b Spinal twist

SPINAL TWIST

Grasp the foot from the instep with both your hands, fingers on the dorsal side and thumbs on the plantar aspect – the web between the thumb and the index finger against the spinal reflex. When working the right foot, the right hand will be positioned close to the ankle joint, and vice versa on the left foot. This hand is also the support hand. The working hand will execute the twisting action. The two hands should be used as a unit, keeping all the fingers together and the hands touching.

Keep the support hand very steady and twist the foot with the working hand 'up and down'. The support hand must remain completely stationary. Then move both hands forward slightly and repeat the twisting action. Continue this movement (grip, twist, reposition, grip, twist and reposition) until you reach the neck reflex area at the base of the big toe. Do not twist both hands at the same time. This technique can be practised on a cloth in order to master the action performed by the two hands as a single unit.

The spine

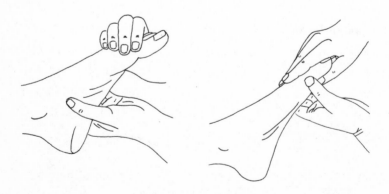

Fig. 28 Spine Grip H

GRIP H

The support hand is held in the standard support grip. Cup the instep towards the heel of the foot in the palm of the working hand, pulling the foot down towards you with the support hand until the toes are in a more horizontal position. The thumb is left free to execute the rotating thumb technique on the medial side of the foot, with the four fingers supporting on the lateral side of the foot.

As the spine represents the midline of the body, the reflex is found in the same position on both feet. The reflex area on each foot corresponds to half the spine. The spine reflex runs the length of the curve on the medial aspect of the foot. Treating this reflex will activate blood flow to the spine, loosen vertebrae and muscles in this area, and have a stimulating effect on the entire body by invigorating activity of the nerve impulses. This will also stimulate the central nervous system.

Begin with the spinal twist to loosen the spine. Repeat this on the other foot. If the foot is tense it may be necessary to repeat a few times. This is a very effective tension reducer enjoyed by most. It may happen from time to time that you will hear a clicking sound when performing this technique. This may signify misalignments in the spine being corrected.

Therapist position: To execute this grip effectively, you must be seated in such a way as to be able to swivel in your seat and face the foot to be worked on at an angle from the medial side. Your shoulders should be relaxed, your spine straight, elbows down and your arms loosely at your sides. Your feet should be placed squarely on the ground, slightly apart. Remember to keep eye contact with your patient.

To work the spinal reflex, use Grip H. Start at the tip of the heel and work up the spine to the toes. The rotating thumb should be used effectively to loosen each vertebra. It is imperative to work this area thoroughly and, more often than not, tight areas will be found here. When bending the foot towards you with the support hand, you can 'see' the shape of the spine quite clearly. Work next to and up against the bony structure on the instep – first along the coccyx and clearly defined sacral curve, then over the bladder reflex and along the navicular bone, from where you will follow the metatarsals. Be careful not to work directly on the bone, but slightly under it, using it as your guideline instead. Pay special attention when you reach the base of the big toe, as the seven cervical vertebrae start here and continue to the tip of the toe. Your support hand will change when reaching the metatarsalphalange joint at the base of the big toe, supporting the toe between the thumb, placed on the plantar aspect of the foot, and the index and middle fingers from above with the four fingers pointing towards the ankle.

Therapist position: When changing to Grip H, change your seating position at the same time to face the feet directly. Keep your arms loosely at your sides with your elbows down. Keep your shoulders relaxed, your spine straight and your feet placed squarely on the ground, slightly apart. Remember to keep eye contact with your patient.

Outer Body – Lateral Foot

Knee, hip, elbow and shoulder

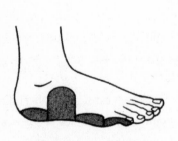

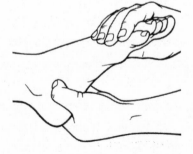

Fig. 29a Knee, hip, elbow
and shoulder

Fig. 29b Grip H

GRIP H

The support hand is held in the standard support grip. Cup the instep towards the heel of the foot in the palm of the working hand, pulling the foot down towards you with the support hand until the toes are in a more horizontal position. The thumb is left free to execute the rotating thumb technique on the lateral side of the foot, with the four fingers supporting on the medial side of the foot.

The four reflexes, namely the knee, hip, elbow and shoulder, run the length of the lateral side of the foot. The first two can be found below the waistline, with the last two above. The waistline is demarcated by the protrusion of the fifth metatarsal, where it joins with the cuboid bone.

The knee reflex extends across the heel area, followed by the hip reflex, which covers the largest area. This reflex covers an oblong shape ending in line with the fourth toe and gall bladder meridian point. This area may be puffy, which could indicate hip weakness or posture problems associated with the lower back and gall bladder meridian.

The elbow reflex can be found from the waistline through to the diaphragm reflex. The shoulder reflex corresponds to the area alongside the ball of the foot, extending to just below the fifth toe on both the plantar and dorsal aspects. Note: As part of the bladder meridian, which traverses the vertebrae and spine in the entire back, runs along this section of the foot, this is also an excellent referral reflex for the spine.

Use Grip H as with the spinal reflex, but with opposite working and supporting hands. Begin at the knee reflex at the back of the heel and work along the edge of the foot towards the toes. When working the hip reflex, move up the dorsal side of the foot until in line with the fourth toe and the gall bladder meridian. Move back to the edge of the foot once the hip reflex has been covered and continue working in line with the metatarsals and distal phalange to the base of the little toe. Repeat the same procedure on the other foot.

Therapist position: Face the feet directly, with your arms kept loosely at your sides. Keep your shoulders relaxed, your spine straight and your elbows down. Your feet should be placed squarely on the ground, slightly apart. Remember to keep eye contact with your patient.

Circulation and Breasts – Dorsal Foot and Posterior Leg

Breasts, circulation and kidney/bladder meridians

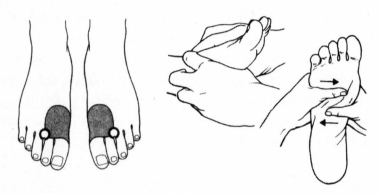

Fig. 30a Breast and circulation   Fig. 30b Finger technique 4

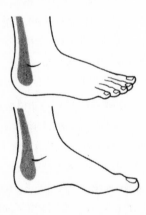

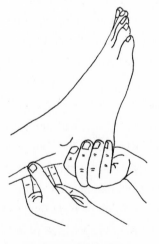

Fig. 31a Kidney/bladder meridians   Fig. 31b Pinch technique

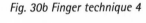

FINGER TECHNIQUE 4

Use both hands. Place your hands on opposite sides of the foot, thumbs on the plantar aspect forming the support and four fingers on the dorsal side. During the first part of this technique, the eight fingers are the working tools, massaging with a slow and smooth rotating pressure. During the second stage of this technique, the thumbs perform a criss-cross movement on the plantar aspect of the foot.

PINCH TECHNIQUE

The support hand cups the foot at the ankle, while the working hand locates the Achilles tendon at the back of the heel and moves up and down the tendon, 'pinching' it gently between the thumb and index finger. (This is used to stimulate the kidney and bladder meridians.)

The breast reflexes are found on the dorsal aspect of the feet in line with the big and second toes, corresponding to the same range as the ball of the foot on the plantar side. The special circulation reflexes are situated on the dorsal aspect of the feet on the web between the second and third toes.

The kidney and bladder meridians run up the back of the ankle along opposite sides of the Achilles tendon. Pressure here will help clear any congestion in the lower sections of these meridians and thus the related organs.

As this is part of the winding down stage of the treatment, herbal cream or aromatic oils are used to facilitate smooth and easy movements. This also helps to relax the patient and leave them with good memories, which is particularly important if the treatment has been sensitive.

The best way to work on these reflexes is to use the eight fingers simultaneously, as in Finger Technique 4, starting at the groin area corresponding with the ankle joint. Exert deep, rotating pressure with the fingers, massaging smoothly and slowly down the foot towards the toes. Apply extra pressure to the special circulation points in the webs between the second and third toes. Repeat this procedure a few times. Then use the criss-cross movement with the thumbs on the plantar aspect of the foot. At this stage you can improvise by adding your own creativity, but ensure that the area is massaged thoroughly.

Stimulation of the kidney and bladder meridians is incorporated into the massage begun with Finger Technique 4. Locate the Achilles tendon at the back of the ankle and apply the Pinch Technique, moving up and down the tendon. This area may be extremely sensitive so proceed with care and ensure that your fingers are moist with cream or oil. Repeat the above procedures and techniques on the other foot.

Therapist position: Face the feet directly, with your arms kept loosely at your sides. Keep your shoulders relaxed, your spine straight and your elbows down. Your feet should be placed squarely on the ground, slightly apart. Remember to keep eye contact with your patient.

Relaxation Technique

Solar plexus – deep breathing

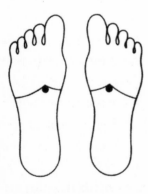

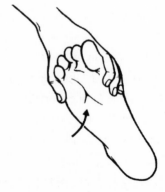

Fig. 32a Solar plexus   *Fig. 32b Finding the solar plexus reflex*

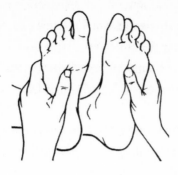

Fig. 33 Solar plexus deep breathing

SOLAR PLEXUS DEEP BREATHING TECHNIQUE

Grasp the feet from the lateral side of the foot in both hands – the left foot in the right hand and the right foot in the left hand, fingers on the dorsal side, thumbs on the plantar aspects. Place the tips of the thumbs on the solar plexus reflex. Ask the patient to lean back, close their eyes and breathe as slowly and deeply as is comfortable for them. Apply pressure to the reflex while the patient is inhaling and release pressure while exhaling. Do not lose contact with the reflex.

The solar plexus has been termed the 'nerve switchboard' of the body, as it is the main storage area for stress. Furthermore kidney meridian point 1 is also found on this reflex, so treatment of this point will have a positive impact on blood pressure. Applying pressure to this reflex will always bring about a feeling of relaxation.

To locate the solar plexus reflex, grasp the dorsal side of the foot in the metatarsal area and squeeze gently. A depression will appear on the plantar aspect of the foot at the centre of the diaphragm line – the midpoint of the base of the ball of the foot. This is the solar plexus reflex/kidney meridian point 1.

This technique is applied to both feet simultaneously. Pressure applied to this reflex is used as a relaxation technique to complete the treatment.

However, it can be used at any time during treatment, for instance to help the patient relax afterwards when a reflex was particularly sensitive, or to pause during the treatment when talking to your patient. Note that for the latter you would merely apply light pressure to the reflex, rather than stimulating it by following the breathing patterns.

Repeat the technique a number of times until your patient is relaxed and at ease. Following treatment, the patient should sit quietly and relax for a few minutes.

Therapist position: Face the feet directly, with your arms kept loosely at your sides. Keep your shoulders relaxed, your spine straight and your elbows down. Your feet should be placed squarely on the ground, slightly apart. Instead of keeping eye contact with the patient, you should observe their breathing by keeping an eye on their chest movements. This will indicate when to apply or release pressure to the reflex.

Step-By-Step Treatment Sequence

The treatment sequence is divided into the same main areas as mentioned in 'Mapping the Feet'.

- Head and neck area = the toes;
- Thoracic area = the ball;
- Abdominal area = the arch;
- Pelvic area = the heel;
- Reproductive area = the ankles;
- Spine = the medial foot;
- Outer body = the lateral foot;
- Circulation = the dorsal foot.

Do not forget – the feet are worked on alternately, from toe to heel, mainly organ by organ.

Easy Reference Treatment Procedure

Relaxation techniques

1 Achilles tendon stretch
2 Ankle rotation
3 Side to side
4 Loosen ankle
5 Wringing the foot
6 Rotate all toes

Head and neck area – the toes and meridians

- Sinus from big toe to small toe – Grip A
- Pituitary gland – Grip B or C

- Brain matter, neck, eyes and ears – Grip B
- Sides and dorsal aspect of toes (the meridians) – Finger Technique 1, Grip D
- Eustachian tubes, chronic eyes and ears – Grip A
- Upper lymphatic system – Finger Technique 2

Thoracic area – the ball

- Bronchi, lungs, and heart – Grip A
- Thyroid, parathyroid and oesophagus – Grip E
- Diaphragm – Grip F

Abdominal area – the arch

- Liver, gall bladder – Grip G
- Stomach, pancreas, duodenum, spleen – Grip G
- Small intestine, ileo-caecal valve, appendix, large intestine, rectum, anus – Grip G
- Kidneys, adrenal glands, ureters – Grip G
- Bladder – Grip H

Pelvic area

- Pelvis and sciatic nerve – Knead technique

Reproductive area

- Uterus/prostate/ovaries/testes – Grip H
- Fallopian tubes/vas deferens – Finger technique 3

Spine – medial foot

- Spinal twist – Loosen the spine
- Spine from heel to toe – Grip H

Outer Body – lateral foot

- Knee, hip, elbow, shoulder – Grip H

Circulation, breasts – dorsal foot/posterior leg

- Circulation and breast area – Finger technique 4
- Bladder and kidney meridians – Pinch technique

Relaxation technique

- Solar plexus – Deep breathing

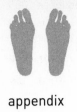

the vacuflex system

Through the sophistication of modern technology, but without losing the human touch, the Vacuflex System maximizes the body's own healing potential, by combining, in one treatment, two of the world's most ancient and powerful methods of holistic practice, reflexology and meridian therapy. The Vacuflex System combines a vacuum boot therapy stimulating the reflexes, together with a vacuum cup treatment of the acupuncture points of the meridians.

Vacuum therapy is acknowledged as an ancient treatment, having been practised since primitive times when animal horns were used as cups. Cups made from burnt clay were discovered in ancient Mesopotamia. In Greece these cups were made of bronze, while other examples have been found constructed of brass, porcelain and glass. The Vacuflex cups, referred to as 'pads' are made of silicone. Needles, lasers, finger pressure or suction cups placed on specific meridian points stimulate related nerves, which transmit electrical impulses to the spinal cord and brain. The suction pressure increases the flow of blood and oxygen to congested areas, causing toxic stagnation to disperse. The pressure also encourages tissue and muscle regeneration by stimulating blood supply and nutrients to the affected area.

Possible the most remarkable feature of the Vacuflex System is the dis-
colouration appearing on the plantar and dorsal regions of the feet
when the boots are removed, and the first stage of the treatment has
taken place – that of stimulating the reflexes and the meridians in the
feet. This is caused by the pressure of the boots and highlights areas of
reflex and meridian congestion. The colours remain for approximately
30 seconds during which time the therapist can 'read' and 'assess' what
is reflected.

This visual impression is of the utmost importance in firstly, tracing the
disease pathways; secondly, it will monitor the changes in the colour
patterns as elimination takes place with each treatment. The colours
that appear are red, blue, yellow and white.

These colours are a measure of the thermal energy of the body showing heat or lack thereof, reflecting the energy conditions as they are at
that present moment in time. The colour red indicates high acid
deposits; the colour blue appears when the body is in acute pain or
there are stresses in the organs. The yellow appears where mucus accu-
mulates in the body and the white appears where there is a chronic or
long-term condition or a candida (yeast) infection. Patients with lower
resistance will often have the most colourful feet; however, chronic
conditions show very pale, confirming a lack of oxygen in the cellular
levels. The lack of colour is in fact an indication that these patients are
lacking in heat – Chi.

Normal body temperature is 98.4° F (with a range from 97 to 99
degrees) and 36.9° C (with a range from 36.1 to 37.2 degrees). This temperature is maintained by an exact adjustment between heat produced
and heat lost by the body. The body's heat-regulating centre is in the
hypothalamus and it acts like a thermostat due to its extreme sensitivity to the temperature of the blood passing through it. The temperature
of the blood depends on the amount and quality of fuel (food) that is
consumed. Heat is produced directly by metabolic activities in the

skeletal muscles and liver. The glycogen stored in the liver is converted into usable glucose and oxidized, resulting in heat (thermal) production (wood – generates fire).

When confronted with a patient showing very pale feet after removal of the boots – it is important to be aware of the possibility of deep-rooted conditions. The patient might be taking strong tissue-blocking medication, such as cortisone. Another cause for paleness of the feet is a tendency towards a severe yeast infection. Usually, after a few treatments, colours will start to appear on the reflexes of the feet. This is directly as a result of increased oxygen levels in the body brought about by the treatments of the Vacuflex System. This is a sign of the reflexes and consequently their corresponding organs being revitalized.

The case assessments that follow clearly show that a reflexologist cannot 'diagnose' congestions according to the 'simplicity' of the reflexology chart but has to take many levels of consideration into account.

CASE 1

A female patient showed on her feet congestion in her sigmoid colon reflex. Having noted this, it was not 'diagnosed' or suggested that she had any problems in this area. Rather, the therapist placed her hands over the corresponding area of the patient's body, covering the area on the front and back, asking if she was aware of any upsets in this region on her body. At first nothing was noted or remembered. At her next visit, the congestion displayed on her foot as a blue spot (blue being the colour of an acute stress-related problem) and appeared on the other foot, suggesting that the blockage had moved to the other side of her body. As a result it was discovered that a hormone replacement plaster was causing tissues of her buttock some stress, and it had indeed been moved from one side of her body to the other in between the two treatments. This example clearly shows that a diagnosis is not possible. There is no way of knowing from her reflexes in the feet and the congestions reflected that her hormone replacement plaster was causing some bodily upset. What we assess is changes in the thermal levels taking place. This is not to say that anyone using a hormone replacement plaster will automatically suffer from some form of bodily stress and upset. Each person is an individual and responds differently to internal and external influences.

CASE 2

A male patient, suffering from exhaustion after a bypass operation, consistently showed a blue patch in the medial lower part of his foot, which relates to the reflex for the lower back/rectum region. As with the previous case study, hands were placed on the corresponding area of his body, and on asking if any form of stress was experienced in this section, the answer was 'no', other than a slight occasional irritation. As a follow up to his bypass operation, he underwent a routine x-ray of the area, which revealed that a metal clamp stitch had been left inside his body. It was removed and the blue (acute) patch on his foot disappeared.

Neither the Vacuflex System nor reflexology has the capacity to give a diagnosis – however the Vacuflex System clearly indicates the area of thermal changes and therefore creates an assessment tool that can benefit the healing process.

The second stage of Vacuflex treatment is the application of suction pads on the acupuncture points along the meridians, using the sections of the arms and lower legs; other parts of the meridians can also be used. As soon as pressure is exerted at the acupuncture point, the meridian is stimulated and any blockage in the energy flow along the pathway is dispersed.

references

Chapter 1

1   Harry Bond Bressler, *Zone Therapy*, p 29
2   Christine Issel, *Reflexology: Art, Science and History*, pp 30–1
3   Ibid, p 35
4   Ibid, pp 24–5
5   Michelle Arnot, *Foot Notes*, pp 8–9
6   Ibid, p 21
7   Ibid, p 28
8   Ibid, p 30
9   *Reflexology: Art, Science and History*, pp 54–5
10 Ibid, p 63
11 Ibid, pp 120–1
12 Ann Gillanders, *Reflexology – The Ancient Answer to Modern Ailments*, p 13

Chapter 2

1   Harriet Beinfield and Efrem Korngold, *Between Heaven and Earth: A Guide to Chinese Medicine*, 1991, p 30

2   Daniel Reid, *Guarding the Three Treasures*, p 22

3   Ibid, p 16

4   Daniel Reid, *The Tao of Health Sex and Longevity*, p 6

5   *Guarding the Three Treasures*, pp 16, 20

6   Daniel Reid, *The Shambhala Guide to Traditional Chinese Medicine*, p 23

7   *Between Heaven and Earth*, p 5

8   Richard Gerber, *Vibrational Medicine*, p 178

9   *Between Heaven and Earth*, p 31

10   Ted Kaptchuk, *The Web That Has No Weaver*, p 45

11   Kim Le, PhD, *The Simple Path to Health*, p 24

12   *Guarding the Three Treasures*, p 4

13   *The Simple Path to Health*, p 24

14   Jason Elias and Katherine Ketcham, *The Five Elements of Self-Healing*, p 278

15   *Guarding the Three Treasures*, p 4

16   Philippa McKinley, 'Secrets of the Life Force', *Here's Health* magazine, January 1991

17   D and J Lawson-Wood, *The Five Elements of Acupuncture and Chinese Massage*, pp 70, 20

18   Philippa McKinley, 'Secrets of the Life Force' , *Here's Health* magazine, January 1991

19   Robert Becker, MD, and Gary Seldon, *The Body Electric*, pp 79–80

20   Lyall Watson, *Beyond Supernature*, pp 92–7

21   John Davidson, *Subtle Energy*, p 19

22   Ibid, p 122–3

23   Lyall Watson, *Supernature II*, p 105

24   *Beyond Supernature*, p 102

25   *Guarding the Three Treasures*, p 25

26   *Between Heaven and Earth*, p 49

27   Chee Soo, *The Taoist Ways of Healing*, p 24

28   Richard Hyatt, *Chinese Herbal Medicine*, pp 30–1

29   Ilza Veith, *The Yellow Emperor's Classic of Internal Medicine*, p 14

30   *Chinese Herbal Medicine*, pp 30–1

31   *Between Heaven and Earth*, p 29

32   *The Shambhala Guide to Traditional Chinese Medicine*, pp 22–3

33   *Guarding the Three Treasures*, p 32

34   Ibid, pp 32–3

35   *Chinese Herbal Medicine*, p 31

36   Ibid, p 31

37   *The Taoist Ways of Healing*, p 28

38   *The Shambhala Guide to Traditional Chinese Medicine*, p 27

39   *The Simple Path to Health*, p 16

40   *The Shambhala Guide to Traditional Chinese Medicine*, p 27

41   *The Yellow Emperor's Classic of Internal Medicine*, p 19

42   Dianne M Connelly, *Traditional Acupuncture: The Law of the Five Elements*, p 16

43   *Vibrational Medicine*, pp 178–9

44   Ibid, pp 180–1

45   Liu Yanchi, *The Essential Book of Traditional Chinese Medicine*, p 54

46   *The Shambhala Guide to Traditional Chinese Medicine*, p 28

47   *The Essential Book of Traditional Chinese Medicine*, p 18

48   Ibid, p 25

49   Wataru Ohashi and Tom Monte, *Reading the Body*, p 10

50   *The Essential Book of Traditional Chinese Medicine*, p 166

51   Ibid, p 166

52   *The Simple Path to Health*, p 27

53   *The Essential Book of Traditional Chinese Medicine*, p 24

54   Robert Svoboda and Arnie Lade, *Tao and Dharma*, p 24

55   Elson M Haas, *Staying Healthy with the Seasons*, p 28

56   *Vibrational Medicine*, p 182

57   *The Web That Has No Weaver*, p 106

58   Ibid, p 106

Chapter 3

1   Laura Norman with Thomas Cowan, *Feet First*, p 130
2   Robert Becker, MD, and Gary Seldon, *The Body Electric*, p 292
3   E Cheraskin, WM Ringsdorf Jr and Arline Brecher, *Psychodietetics*
4   Alvin Toffler, *Future Shock*
5   *Critical Condition – Healthcare in America*, Tuberose Publishing

Chapter 4

1   *The Five Elements of Acupuncture and Chinese Massage*, p 40
2   *Traditional Acupuncture: The Law of the Five Elements*, p 27
3   Ibid, p 25
4   *The Yellow Emperor's Classic of Internal Medicine*, p 109
5   Janet Riddle, *Anatomy and Physiology Applied to Nursing*, p 51
6   *Traditional Acupuncture: The Law of the Five Elements*, pp 51–2, 63–4
7   Ibid, p 63
8   *The Web That Has No Weaver*, pp 56–7
9   John F Thie, *Touch For Health*, p 96
10 Ibid, p 98
11 Ibid, p 100
12 Ibid, p 102
13 Ibid, p 104
14 Ibid, p 106
15 Ibid, p 108
16 *The Yellow Emperor's Classic of Internal Medicine*, p 133
17 Ibid, p 139
18 *Traditional Acupuncture: The Law of the Five Elements*, p 54
19 *The Web That Has No Weaver*, pp 57–68
20 *Touch For Health*, p 36
21 Ibid, p 38
22 Ibid, p 40

23 *The Yellow Emperor's Classic of Internal Medicine*, p 133

24 *The Web That Has No Weaver*, p 58

25 Ibid, pp 58–9

26 *Touch For Health*, p 44

27 Ibid, p 46

28 Ibid, p 48

29 Ibid, p 50

30 *The Yellow Emperor's Classic of Internal Medicine*, p 133

31 Ibid, p 139

32 Iona Marsaa-Teegurden, *Handbook of Acupressure*, p 12

33 *The Web That Has No Weaver*, p 54; *Handbook of Acupressure*, p 16

34 *The Web That Has No Weaver*, p 54

35 *Touch For Health*, p 52

36 *The Yellow Emperor's Classic of Internal Medicine*, p 133

37 *Handbook of Acupressure*, p 12

38 *Touch For Health*, p 54

39 Ibid, p 56

40 *Staying Healthy with the Seasons*

41 *The Yellow Emperor's Classic of Internal Medicine*, p 133

42 *Handbook of Acupressure* p 20; *The Web That Has No Weaver*, p 68; *Traditional Acupuncture: The Law of the Five Elements*, p 78

43 *Touch For Health*, p 58

44 Ibid, p 60

45 Ibid, p 62

46 *The Yellow Emperor's Classic of Internal Medicine*, p 133

47 Ibid, p 139

48 *The Web That Has No Weaver*, pp 62–3

49 *Traditional Acupuncture: The Law of the Five Elements*, p 77

50 *Handbook of Acupressure*, p 22

51 *Touch For Health*, p 64

52 Ibid, p 66

53 Ibid, p 68

54 *Handbook of Acupressure*, p 25

55 *Touch For Health*, p 70

56 Ibid, p 72

57 Ibid, p 74

58 Ibid, p 76

59 *The Yellow Emperor's Classic of Internal Medicine*, p 133

60 *Handbook of Acupressure*, p 26

61 Ibid, p 26

62 *Touch For Health*, p 78

63 Ibid, p 80

64 Ibid, p 82

65 Ibid, p 84

66 Ibid, p 86

67 *The Yellow Emperor's Classic of Internal Medicine*, p 133

68 *Handbook of Acupressure*, p 22

69 Ibid, p 28

70 *The Web That Has No Weaver*, pp 66–7

71 *Touch For Health*, p 28

72 Ibid, p 90

73 *The Yellow Emperor's Classic of Internal Medicine*, p 133

74 *The Web That Has No Weaver*, pp 59–60

75 *Handbook of Acupressure*, p 30

76 *The Web That Has No Weaver*, p 60; *Handbook of Acupressure*, p 30

77 *Touch For Health*, p 92

78 Ibid, p 94

79 *The Web That Has No Weaver*, p 78

80 Yoshio Manaka, MD, and Ian A Urquhart, PhD, *The Layman's Guide to Acupuncture*, p 73

81 Mark Seem, PhD, with Joan Kaplan, *Bodymind Energetics*, p 33

82 Chinese Traditional Medical College, *Anatomical Charts of the Acupuncture Points and 14 Meridians*, p 51; *The Web That Has No Weaver*, p 104

83 Jorgen Frydenlund, *Meridianlaren*, Forlaget Alterna

84 *Touch For Health*, p 34

85 *Bodymind Energetics*, p 33

86 Chinese Traditional Medical College, p 55; *The Web That Has No Weaver*, p 107

87 *Touch For Health*, p 32

Chapter 5

1 Omraam Mikhael Aivanhov, *The Zodiac, Key to Man and to the Universe*, pp 79–80

2 Ibid, pp 83–9

3 Ibid, pp 92–6

bibliography

Aivanhov, Omraam Mikhael, *The Zodiac, Key to Man and to the Universe*, Editions Prosveta, Fréjus, France, 1986

Arnot, Michelle, *Foot Notes*, Sphere Books Ltd, London, 1982

Ballard, Juliet Brooke, *The Hidden Laws of the Earth*, ARE Press, Virginia Beach, Virginia, 1986

Bayley, Doreen, *Reflexology Today*, Thorsons, New York, 1986

Becker, Robert, MD, and Seldon, Gary, *The Body Electric*, Quill, William Morrow, New York, 1985

Blofeld, John, *Taoism – The Quest For Immortality*, Unwin Paperbacks, London, 1979

Bressler, Harry Bond, *Zone Therapy*, Health Research, Mokelumne Hill, California, 1971

Brown, Guy, *The Energy of Life*, HarperCollins, London, 1999

Burr, Harold Saxton, *Blueprint for Immortality*, The CW Daniel Company Limited, Saffron Walden, 1972

Byers, Dwight C, *Better Health with Foot Reflexology*, Ingham Publishing, St Petersburg, Florida, 1986

Cheraskin, E, and Ringsdorf Jr, WM, with Brecher, Arline, *Psychodietetics*, Bantam Books, New York, 1985

Chinese Traditional Medical College of Shanghai and Chinese Traditional Research Institute of Shanghai, *Anatomical Charts of*

the Acupuncture Points and 14 Meridians, Shanghai People's
    Publishing House, 1976

Chopra, Deepak, MD, *Perfect Health*, Bantam Books, Transworld
    Publishers, London, 1990

Connelly, Dianne M, PhD, MAC, *Traditional Acupuncture: The Law of
    the Five Elements*, The Centre for Traditional Acupuncture Inc,
    Columbia, Maryland, 1989

Copen, Bruce, PhD, DLitt, *Magic of the Aura*, Academic Publications,
    Haywards Heath, 1976

Davidson, John, *Subtle Energy*, The CW Daniel Company Limited,
    Saffron Walden, 1987

Eden, Donna, *Energy Medicine*, JP Tarcher/Putman, New York, 1998

Fast, Julius, *You and Your Feet*, Pelham Books, London, 1971

Fitzgerald, William H, and Bowers, Edwin F, *Zone Therapy*, Health
    Research, Mokelumne Hill, California, 1917

Frydenlund, Jorgen, *Meridianlaren*, Forlaget Alterna

Gerber, Richard, MD, *Vibrational Medicine for the 21st Century*, W
    Morrow and Company, New York, 2000

Gillanders, Ann, *Reflexology – The Ancient Answer to Modern
    Ailments*, Gillanders, 1987

Goosman-Legger, Astrid, *Zone Therapy Using Foot Massage*, The CW
    Daniel Company Limited, Saffron Walden, 1983

Gore, Anya, *Reflexology*, Optima, London, 1990

Grinberg, Avi, *Holistic Reflexology*, Thorsons, Wellingborough, 1989

Hall, Nicola M, *Reflexology – A Patient's Guide*, Thorsons,
    Wellingborough, 1986

Hall, Nicola M, *Reflexology – A Way to Better Health*, Pan Books,
    London, 1988

Holford, Patrick, 'Population Protection', *Here's Health* magazine,
    August 1989

Holford, Patrick, *Optimum Nutrition Bible*, Piatkus Books, London,
    2004

Ingham, Eunice D, *Stories the Feet Can Tell Thru Reflexology*, Ingham
    Publishing, St Petersburg, Florida, 1938, 1951

Issel, Christine, *Reflexology: Art, Science and History*, New Frontier
    Publishing, Sacramento, 1990

Kaptchuk, Ted J, OMD, *The Web That Has No Weaver*, Congden and
    Weed, New York, 1983

Kunz, Kevin, and Barbara, *The Complete Guide to Foot Reflexology*,
    Thorsons, Wellingborough, 1982

Lakhovsky, Georges, *The Secret of Life*, The Noontide Press, USA, 1935,
    1992

Lawson-Wood, D, and J, *The Five Elements of Acupuncture and
    Chinese Massage*, Health Science Press, Devon, 1985

Lewith, George, MD and Kenyon, Julian, MD, *Clinical Ecology*,
    Thorsons, Wellingborough, 1985

Marsaa Teeguarden, Iona, *Handbook of Acupressure II*, Ginseng du
    Foundation, 1981

MacDonald, Alexander, *Acupuncture – From Ancient Art to Modern
    Medicine*, Unwin, London, 1982

Mackereth, Peter A, and Tiran, Denise, *Clinical Reflexology*, Churchill
    Livingstone, London, 2002

Majhisttagenmalm, *Zonterapi og Urtemeduim*, Komma Helse

Manaka, Yoshio, MD, and Urquhart, Ian A, PhD, *The Layman's Guide to
    Acupuncture*, Weatherhill, New York, 1972

Mann, Felix, *Acupuncture*, Pan Books, London, 1971

Manning, Clark A, *Bioenergetic Medicines – East and West*, North
    Atlantic Books, Berkeley, 1988

Marquardt, Hanne, *Reflex Zone Therapy of the Feet*, Thorsons,
    Wellingborough, 1983

Mason, Keith, *Medicine for the 21st Century*, Element Books,
    Shaftesbury, 1992

McKinley, Philippa, 'Secrets of the Life Force', *Here's Health* magazine,
    January 1991

Nightingale, Michael, *Acupuncture*, Optima, London, 1987

Norman, Laura, with Cowan, Thomas, *Feet First*, Simon and Schuster
    Inc, New York, 1988

Nuland, Sherwin B, *How We Live*, Vintage, London, 1998

Pike, Geoff, *The Power of Ch'I*, Bay Books, Sydney, 1980

Reid, Daniel, *Traditional Chinese Medicine*, Shambhala, London, 1996

Riddle, Janet, *Anatomy and Physiology Applied to Nursing*, Churchill
    Livingstone, Edinburgh, 1985

Russel, Lewis, and Hardy, Bob, *Healthy Feet*, Optima, London, 1988

Seem, Mark, PhD, with Kaplan, Joan, *Bodymind Energetics*, Thorsons,
    Wellingborough, 1987

Sills, Franklyn, *The Polarity Process*, Element Books, Shaftesbury, 1989

Soo, Chee, *The Taoist Ways of Healing*, Aquarian Press,
    Wellingborough, 1986

Stanway, Dr Andrew, *Alternative Medicine – A Guide to Natural
    Therapies*, Penguin Books, London, 1982

Thie, John F, *Touch For Health*, TH Enterprises, Pasadena, California,
    1973

Toffler, Alvin, *Future Shock*, The Bodley Head, London, 1975

Veith, Ilza, *The Yellow Emperor's Classic of Internal Medicine*,
    University of California Press, Berkeley, 1972

Wagner, Franz, PhD, *Reflex Zone Massage*, Thorsons, Wellingborough,
    1987

Walker, Kristine, *Hand Reflexology*, Quay Books, 2002

Watson, Lyall, *Supernature*, Coronet Books, London, 1974

Watson, Lyall, *Supernature II*, Sceptre, London, 1987

Watson, Lyall, *Beyond Supernature*, Hodder and Stoughton, London,
    1986

Wills, Pauline, *The Reflexology Manual*, Headline Books, London, 1995

acknowledgements

When walking life's path, gaining knowledge and experience, countless times we will come across footprints showing evidence of others having crossed or shared that same path.

During my many years of private practice, the trust of my patients has given me confidence and encouragement to continue to seek a better understanding of health issues. I would like to thank all my patients for the help they have given in this respect.

Taking reflexology out to a wider audience through teaching has been a great joy, and the incredible feedback and support from students around the world has been of inestimable help and inspiration. I am forever grateful to the many students who have crossed my path, and who have, with their many thought-provoking questions, become my teacher!

My biggest challenge has been the creation of the International Academy of Reflexology and Meridian Therapy, opening campuses around the world, and being involved in the statutory recognition of our profession in South Africa. This has led to having obtained accreditation for our teaching programme by the South African Qualification Authority. Without the amazing support and understanding from some very special people, the programme and its teaching material – and, ultimately, this book – would not have materialized. The teamwork has been phenomenal, and special thanks for sharing my life path and leaving solid footprints as evidence must go to: Louise Moore for her patience in researching, Marian de Jager, Cecilia Salvesen, Dolly Maree, Doret Botha, Tanya Gilman, Salverajan Naidoo, Marinda Nel, Laura Charles, Hoosein Ravat, Brigitte Aubery, Anneliese Potgieter, Elna Steenkamp, Santie Peens, Trudie Putter and Belinda Scrooby for being the great team of school leaders and lecturers in South Africa – believing 100% in the programme; Terralynn Hoskins for taking on the task of introducing the programme into the USA; Geraldine and Keir Giles for their endless support and vision for the programme to enter into the United Kingdom; Dariusz Ruder for opening the school in Poland; Alberto Carnevale-Maffé in Italy, Hanne Damm Corell and Per Bennicke for their hard work in having the programme translated and introduced into my country of birth – Denmark, Sandra Barlavas in Greece, and Emeric Charles for taking the programme into Australia. A special thank you must go to my younger son Thomas for having transformed our programme into interactive CD-ROMs with web-board interaction and a great web site. With the launch of this book, Thomas has created an amazing data-system for taking case studies and linking the information gathered to the content of this book. May our footprints continue together long into the future!

A critical and positive editor is vital for any author to make them feel at ease and Matthew Cory and Susanna Abbott have been there to support, debate and enhance the work – thank you.

As the book is all about understanding old philosophies in a modern context – the greatest acknowledgement must be given to mother Earth for carrying all of our footprints – making us aware of the impact our responsibility towards our individual health has – positively and negatively.

index

THE INTERNATIONAL ACADEMY OF
REFLEXOLOGY
&MERIDIAN
THERAPY

Established 1983

DIPLOMA COURSES IN REFLEXOLOGY AND MERIDIAN THERAPY

Including the study and application, in modular format, of:

- Therapeutic Reflexology
- The principles of Chinese Meridian Philosophies
- Anatomy and Physiology
- Pathology and Pathophysiology

Training is available at licensed campuses of the Academy throughout the world. Qualifications can also be obtained through one of our Distance e-Learning programs, which include interactive CD ROMs and website forum interaction for the theoretical aspects. Practical applications are covered during workshops offered at our various international campuses.

*For a prospectus and further information on the **Vacuflex System** or our unique and comprehensive **Data Management System** software for qualified therapists, contact:*

The International Academy of Reflexology
& Meridian Therapy (Pty) Ltd
PO Box 68283, Bryanston, 2021, South Africa
Tel: +27 11 807 7184   Fax: +27 11 807 7184
E-mail: info@vacuflex.com
Websites: http://www.isrmt.com & http://www.vacuflex.com